£2

Healing in th

OTHER TITLES BY THE SAME AUTHOR

Healing in the 21st Century

Complementary Medicine and Modern Life

JAN DE VRIES

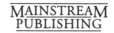
MAINSTREAM
PUBLISHING

EDINBURGH AND LONDON

First published in Great Britain in 2001 by
MAINSTREAM PUBLISHING COMPANY (EDINBURGH) LTD
7 Albany Street
Edinburgh EH1 3UG

ISBN 1 84018 514 7

A catalogue record for this book is available
from the British Library

Typeset in Chancery and Sabon
Printed and bound in Great Britain by
Creative Print and Design Wales

Nobody will ever be able to deny the great achievements of medical science. We need science, however we should never become slaves of science. Science should serve humanity and not the other way around!

Contents

Introduction

All our body cells, the same as microbes, are a form of life. This means that both have their own metabolism; they assimilate nutrients and eliminate waste products. Bacteria, as well as human cells, can be cultivated in a laboratory and as long as the nutrient fluid in which the cells grow contains all the nutrients the cells need and their waste products can be disposed of, these cells stay healthy.

A human being consists of milliards of the tiniest forms of life. Also a human being can only be healthy and procreate when he or she receives the right nutrients and can eliminate waste products. It is a question of input and output, whereby up to a certain point, the output (the excretion of toxins) is even more important than the assimilation of the right nutrients. This is because the accumulation of any kind of waste products, even from the healthiest food, can cause illness.

Although many people do not want to believe this, humans are still part of nature and the laws of nature are the same for all creatures. When bacterial cultures in a laboratory become polluted, the bacteria suffocate in their own dirt and die. When people cannot excrete sufficient waste products, these accumulate somewhere in the body and cause disease.

When the quality of the food is bad and/or when people eat too much, many toxic substances will accumulate in the organism and if the excretory system does not function as well as it should, these substances will accumulate and the person in question will become ill. This is one of the main reasons for the development of our so-called 'civilisation diseases'. Of course the pollution of the environment, too much stress (as DrHans Seleye has pointed out) and other negative factors are part of the problem.

The Laws of Nature

For the earth, for plants, for animals and for all people the laws of nature are always the same. We should try to understand these laws and we should support nature in all its endeavours. All practitioners and patients should understand and follow these natural laws.

Healthy and simple food, as most people ate in former times, as well as fresh air and plenty of exercise are the best guarantees for a long and healthy life. In former times everyone, with the exception of very rich, old or ill people, was used to regular exercise, as their own feet were their most important means of transportation.

Regular bowel movements and a healthy intestinal flora, as well as the optimum functioning of all excretory organs always were and are extremely important.

Of course, in natural medicine things are often not what they should be. However in the case of wrong treatment, because of a lack of knowledge or experience not as much harm is done as in modern, officially recognised, medicine.

It is high time that natural medicine is also officially recognised, as in Germany where there are special schools for healers, the so-called '*heilpraktikers*'. In other countries too all healers should be permitted to practice in a lawful way, while following certain rules. It is a fact that natural healing is far more acceptable and successful than many life and health-endangering treatments of so-called official medicine. In this book and the others in the *Healthcare* series you will find logical explications about the origin of disease and how to prevent and, if still possible, cure your disease, while not taking the risk of becoming ill for the rest of your life through wrong treatment.

CHAPTER ONE

The History of Medicine Seen in a Different Light

Until about a hundred years ago medical knowledge which had been accumulating for thousands of years had been guarded very carefully and every medical student had to know all about the subject. All reputable physicians, beginning with Hippocrates (460–377 BC), were convinced that a profound knowledge of medical history was indispensable for all physicians. Only those who have followed the gradual growth of the art of medicine and who know how much was achieved in the past are able to correctly assess the pros and cons of today's medical science. Pushman, the founder of the school of medical history in Vienna, wrote:

> A physician who neglects to study the history of medicine will often be on the wrong track. He has not learned to avoid the mistakes his predecessors made, because he is used to measure everything with the yardstick of the narrow period of his time.

The medical student of today only rarely hears about the

so very valuable wealth of experience of the past. The Hippocratic oath still means something, but nothing is taught about the successful Hippocratic and other healing methods of olden times. Therefore the medical student gets the impression that these healing ways are old-fashioned and not relevant in our advanced times. Many of them still believe that modrn medicine is the only right thing.

Today one tries to repair damage with the help of technical appliances and chemical-based substances. Many physicians, who apparently do not understand that medicine is not only a science but also an art, are nothing more than highly respected workers in a workshop, which has been installed by the medical and pharmaceutical industry. Unfortunately most of these physicians never learned anything about the art of healing and only know how to repair the damage, not prevent it.

Of course it is possible to be a good physician without learning about medical history. However, if the need arose, for example to free a patient within a short time from terrible pain, that physician would be completely helpless without the medication of the pharmaceutical industry. Unfortunately most painkillers have dangerous side effects and in the long run they can even produce more, and often worse, pain. As mentioned already, physicians in olden times knew many harmless and very effective methods of pain control and treatment. Because of ignorance, and also for financial reasons, these methods are no longer made use of, but the physicians of former times were brilliant in this area. It really is ridiculous to believe that physicians of the past, who lived in the time of Aristotle, Archimedes, Pythagoras, Homer and Plato, were less intelligent than we are.

'Many of them were not beneath us, but even far above us,' as Professor Werner Zabel said. We cannot possibly assume that physicians who were able to heal diseases that in our time are considered to be incurable had less experience or were less knowledgeable then we are.

Of course, in olden times people also made many mistakes, often because of ignorance and superstition, but everyone can learn from their mistakes and from the experience of the old physicians we can learn very much indeed.

In the rest of this chapter you will find useful information on the history of medicine, which is seldom read about and still less will be taught at universities. It is high time to include at least the most important and valuable sections of medical history in the students' curriculums. Then the next generation of physicians will be less helpless, when it comes to the crunch, to really help the patient in a practical way, and without danger.

Medicine in the Course of Time

Besides accidents, sprains and the dislocation of joints, people who lived in prehistoric times often suffered from intoxication, nausea, diarrhoea and gastric problems, as well as from diseases of the eyes, typhoid, malaria or other infectious and parasitic diseases. From the earliest beginnings, mankind suffered from many different diseases. Today we know this because of the findings of a special branch of science called paleopathology, which bases its findings mainly on archaeological excavations.

In the past people saw illness as something alien, caused by evil spirits, or by poison or harmful substances spoiling the body juices. Medicine men, who at the same time were magicians, tried to chase these evil spirits away by using certain rituals; they also cleaned the body by practical means. This was the beginning of 'empirical medicine', which at the time of Hippocrates developed into a real art.

With the help of herbs, thorns and other natural resources, these healers engendered irritations of the skin and haematoma (bleeding under the skin). They made their patients perspire and gave them enemas by pouring water through the hollow stems of plants. They used laxatives and emetics, so that all damaging substances could be discharged.

Through the derivation and the evacuation of disease-provoking substances and the simultaneous exorcism of evil spirits, many patients were healed. (In our time also, the physician who treats body and soul at the same time is the most successful.)

Medicine in Egypt, Greece and Rome

About the medicine of the Aegean period (2000–1000 BC) we know very little. We know only that at the time surgery was already at a very high standard. People attached great importance to hygiene in general and also to personal hygiene. On the island of Crete many relics of very ingenious and first-class sanitary installations have been found.

At the time of Homer, around 800 BC, many campaigns of conquest were being fought. A large number of warriors suffered serious sword wounds and many of them died. Military surgeons were very important persons; these physicians did not use any magic, they only gave practical help. Treatments for internal diseases were not yet known. Only the gods could heal such diseases. For the treatment of the wounds, herbs, leaves and roots, as well as different oils and ointments were used and many plants such as caraway, coriander, fennel, peppermint and sage served for healing as well as for culinary purposes.

In those times people knew war medicine, and religious and magical medicine. There also were travelling doctors, who had usually only primitive means to help their patients and who went from one place to another.

In the temples the priests practised religious medicine. In antiquity such temples were mostly built in the neighbourhood of warm springs. People who wanted to be cured donated money and in ancient Greece more than 400 of these temples were built. Every visitor first had to clean himself by fasting, by vomiting the contents of his stomach, bathing and mental exercises. People often came in crowds to the temples and paid their fees with food, goods or jewellery. During the 'temple sleep' they were cured of their ailments. Partly these cures were due to the right mental attitude of the patient, as they had a great respect for the gods and goddesses. There is no doubt that real feats of healing took place there.

In the beginning practical medicine was only regarded as a craft. Later this was combined with more knowledge and as early as 600 BC people tried to investigate the causes of internal diseases. Now physicians treated diseases, which at the time of Homer it was believed that only the gods could cure.

In tune with the new ways of thinking scientists tried to explain the causes of different diseases on the basis of practical experience and began to classify them. In this way Greek medicine developed more and more into a science. Their specific thinking was the basis for the medicine of today. Unfortunately our modern medicine has become lost in an aimless and dogmatic investigation of details, which no longer has anything to do with the wisdom of the old physicians and their very logical ways of thinking.

On the basis of often-similar observations the physicians of those times came to the conclusion that internal diseases in most cases were due to wrong nutrition in a qualitative and quantitative sense and to mistakes in the physical, as well as the mental, conduct of the patient. Their therapy always included a change of diet, which was then supported by cleaning procedures (laxatives, vomiting, perspiration, bloodletting and so on). They also tried to correct the mistakes in their patient's lifestyle by rearranging his or her daily habits according to natural laws. Special gymnastics were part of the treatment and served also to prevent disease.

The Physicians of Western Greece

The physicians of western Greece were the first representatives of the so-called 'dietetics', the science of the way of living. It was a further development of the philosophy of nature of the ancient Greeks. This science tried to find the natural balance in all the different aspects of life. It not only tried to bring order into the different eating habits of the people, it also tried to re-adjust the balance between work and rest, gymnastics and sports, baths and massages, sleeping and waking, excretions and secretions, stimulating the spirit and the soul.

Health, beauty and vigour as well as intelligence and virtue were Greek ideals, which could be attained by dietetics. Especially in the case of idealistic and ambitious young people this was very successful and there were many sports centres and gymnasiums. Teachers of physical education and coaches not only looked after the training and the fitness of their charges, but they were also eager to teach them the principles of healthy nutrition and lifestyle.

The Medical Schools of Greece

Around the year 500 BC several medical schools developed in Greece. The most important ones were on the island of Kos and on the peninsula of Knidos. The school of Knidos stressed the importance of the local character of the illness. There, where the symptoms of the illness were visible or painful they were suppressed by strong medication, or by a knife or a red-hot iron, by the use of oil and ointments or in some other way. The physicians of Knidos only believed in symptomatic treatment. They did not believe in a general holistic treatment.

On the island of Kos, Hippocrates and his successors had completely different ideas. They were convinced that if someone fell ill, it was not only the part of the body where the symptoms were that was ill, but the whole person. They treated their patients with derivative and excretory measures, which were very successful in the past and had been used by all primitive tribes, as well by the physicians in times of high civilisation.

The Greeks were brilliant observers. Hippocrates observed nature and tried in his therapy to support the natural defence reactions of the body, instead of fighting them. He came to the conclusion that many diseases develop because of a surplus of food, fat, blood and residues of metabolic processes. He taught his pupils that all diseases, which he believed to be the consequence of satiation, could be healed through drainage. Every stage of a therapy was adjusted exactly to the patient's needs and was thoroughly thought out. Every new experience increased the knowledge and the wellbeing of later generations and was written down by Hippocrates and his disciples in the Corpus Hippocrates.

Greek people and also their physicians loved to travel. They not only adapted their ways of treatment from those of their predecessors, but also from those of the Egyptians, the Arabs, Indians, East Asians and especially from the Chinese.

In Kos, as well as in Knidos, gluttony, excessive drinking and an immoral lifestyle were regarded as important causes of disease. Their physicians were convinced that superfluous food residues, which could not be excreted from the body, caused many different diseases.

Illness was due to:

1. Negative influences of the environment, like the weather, the climate, the air, the soil and the water.
2. The wrong lifestyle, wrong food, stress, injuries, the wrong profession for the person in question.
3. The genetic disposition.

Only nature could heal. Hippocrates wrote a book about the art of healing, wherein he said that physicians should never try to treat a patient who could not be helped any more. He had the same understanding for human suffering as Albert Schweitzer and other great thinkers of our time. He also said that the physician should never harm the patient. 'He is the servant of the art [of medicine] and the patient together with the physician should fight the disease!' During the treatment nutrition was very important. Healthy as well as sick people should always eat simple and healthy food.

Hippocratic physicians were convinced that some symptoms of disease, like haemorrhoids and skin rashes, were most often positive signs, which should never be suppressed.

Etiology

The oldest meaning of the word 'etiology' is the science of the deep-lying causes of an illness. Thereby, in medicine one looks first at the cause which is hidden under the most noticeable symptoms. Then one looks again and again for causes at a deeper level, until the original causes are discovered.

For Hippocrates, as well as for many well-known physicians, the etiology was the foundation of every treatment. According to him disease always develops from a combination of many different factors. Hippocrates, 'the best known physician of all time', understood this like nobody else. From him comes the saying: 'Our food will be our medicine, and our medicine will be our food.' Hippocrates understood illness as a biological process, whereby there was a battle going on between the organism of the patient and the disease-provoking toxins or useless substances. He was more interested in the patient and his or her lifestyle than in the disease.

After the death of Hippocrates many of his ideas which were not completely understood were applied in a wrong and different way by the so-called 'Dogmatics', who were looking for a theoretical explanation of his therapeutic success. They were not interested in purging or bloodletting, although essentially these healing methods were extremely important for the Hippocratians. For healthy as well as for ill people strict rules of behaviour were prescribed and the therapeutic freedom of the Hippocratians was lost.

While studying the history of medicine, it will quickly be understood that the methods of healing changed all the time. Every one of these healing systems was officially recognised during a certain period and then rejected again.

As a reaction to the exaggerated dogmatism and the practice of far too many specialists, which was even worse than in our time, the Empirical school developed. These physicians advocated exact knowledge of medical tradition. According to them a good physician should have much experience and powers of observation. He should know the history of medicine and be able to think in a logical way in order to understand the real causes of a disease. The physician should help the patient step by step. The first thing was to introduce a healthy diet, the next step was the choice of the right therapy and remedies and only as a last resort, if there were no other possibilities, the patient should be operated on (cutting) or be treated by burning methods.

These empirical physicians had learned how to recognise the different signs of disease and already knew quite a bit about pharmacology and surgery. However, they could not understand natural relationships and were not interested in the possible underlying causes of disease. The most important thing to them was therapeutic success and they experimented with many different medications.

In the meantime in Alexandria (Egypt) surgery was much developed. Knowledge of specific treatments increased continuoally and some specialists even performed complicated operations on the skull. For the first time in history the Egyptians were permitted to dissect human corpses. The 'golden age' of anatomy had begun. According to the Egyptian physicians illness was due to the congestion (pletora) of the arteries with food residues, whereby the normal functions of the organs were impeded. Because of this, the patients had to fast and many different laxatives and remedies were used to induce vomiting; cupping and burning (cauterisation) were also used. The wrapping of the joints was a beloved way of healing.

Although several well-known Greek physicians from Kos and Knidos went to Egypt, the Egyptian physicians were most influenced by the school of Knidos. Probably the main reason for this was the new developments in the sector of anatomy and surgery.

Other Greek physicians, like Asclepiades of Prusa (91 BC) took up residence in Rome. Medicine in Rome before that time was quite primitive, with the exception of the medicine which was practised by slaves who came from Greece and Egypt; there they had acquired much medical knowledge from the physicians they had worked for.

The Romans knew many herbs and other medical plants. Cabbages in particular were highly regarded and were used for the treatment of many different ailments.

According to Asclepiades diseases developed because of a disturbance of the movements of the atoms in the human body. Like the Empirical physicians, and contrary to the ideas of Hippocrates, he thought that nature could not be of any help.

This was the time when physicians were of the opinion that every process in the human body was purely mechanical. As long as the atoms, the elemental components of which the human body had been made, could move, the organism stayed healthy. If these movements were too slow, they had to be stimulated by rubbing, passive movements (which consisted of motion in a kind of suspended swing) and hydrotherapy. The rubbing was a kind of massage and success depended on the time and intensity of the treatment.

Asclepiades was so fond of hydrotherapy that he was nicknamed 'the cold water physician'. Besides hydrotherapeutic (water) treatments, there were different kinds of diets. He prescribed light, air and music in cases of mental disease. Different plasters, olfactory substances (smelling salts), cupping and now and then bloodletting were also part of his therapeutic programme. He was one of the first physicians to use the fever therapy. Only seldom did he prescribe medication. No work was too much for him and he was in his own way a genius.

These excellent and successful medical achievements unfortunately were soon replaced by easier treatments. The inevitable triumph of mediocrity began with the Methodists. These Methodists tried to find general fundamental formulas, for example the contraction and distension of the body tissues during the different stages of disease. In cases of too much tension, relaxing treatments were used, like bloodletting, warm baths, fasting, vomiting and diuretics or sweat-provoking treatments. In cases of distension, cold water, cold air and a strengthening diet was used.

After some time there was a reaction against the Methodists. The physicians who initiated this new movement were called 'Pneumatists'. For them the quality and quantity of the air we breathe was most important for our health. Air could also enter the body by way of the skin. The Pneumatists knew much about the pulse diagnosis, which was originally used by the Chinese. Their treatments were based mainly on dietetics and physical treatment. They did not like to use much medication. The Pneumatists prescribed lifestyle and nutrition according to the age and the type of person; real medical intervention was rather rare. However it is interesting to know that the physicians of that period prescribed bloodletting not only in the usual ways, but they also encouraged nosebleeding.

Out of the school of the Pneumatists, who looked for the best in all the different schools of medicine, the school of the Eclectists developed. These tried to combine the ideas of Hippocrates with those of Knidos, Alexandria and the Dogmatics. However, this turned out to be impossible, because of the rigid attitude of many physicians and scientists, who regarded the old and well-tried healing methods as being meaningless. They preferred to declare that many diseases were incurable anyway!

Galen

Galen (129–99 BC) brought a renaissance of the healing methods of Hippocrates. He wrote 20 volumes about the between connections many different diseases. His books also contained much practical advice. Galen considered the prevention of disease as just as important as the treatments. Also for him the etiology, the actual causes of disease, was extremely important.

He observed how the organism, with the help of fever, inflammation, perspiration, abscesses and pus, removed toxins so that the disease could heal. Fever was a healing reaction which took place when the arteries were blocked because of inflammation or because there was too much putrefaction in the intestines.

With the help of an inflammation the organism tried to get rid of toxins in the form of serum (lymphatic fluids), pus or waste materials. The most important task of the physician was to support these cleaning efforts of the organism. Therefore Galen, just like Hippocrates, insisted that the physician should learn as much as possible about the healing methods of empirical medicine. Galen and other successors of the Hippocratic school were convinced that most diseases were due to wrong living habits. Also strong passions, like too much ambition, avarice, irritation, anger, fear and so on could cause illness.

Although Galen in his heart was a follower of Hippocrates, who completely agreed with Aristotle,when he said: 'Nature never does anything without a reason', he was also a scientist, an explorer and an author.

As a physician he had much experience, he was a good surgeon and physiotherapist. He had his own theories about the blood circulation and was very much interested in anatomy and in the localisation of the different diseases.

In his opinion medicine was not only an art, but also a science and although his experiments were still full of mistakes and quite primitive, our modern medicine is indebted to him.

After the death of Galen medicine practically came to a standstill. This status quo continued almost till the end of the fifteenth century. Just as in the school of Knidos, physicians of this period had the tendency to arrange all diseases according to a systematic pattern and the treatment of these corresponded to specific rules. Under the semblance of exactitude, medicine again had fallen into a rigid dogmatism. Like today, medicine deviated more and more from the practical truth and often failed when treating patients.

Galen had noticed that people wanted remedies. Pharmacology and the preparation of drugs became ever more important. The first period of the Middle Ages was called the Period of the Monks. In times of the Pest, for example from 535–1179, monasteries were the last refuge for many patients. The special herbs and medical treatments of Hildegard of Bingen are still known and lately have come back into fashion. She was the abbess of a convent; she helped many patients with her herbs so that they would be able to resist the 'bad influence of the devil'.

When in the year 1130 the monks were forbidden to practise medicine, the first schools of medicine were opened in Salerno and Montpelier. There Greek medicine was taught in combination with the healing methods of the Arabs. Even women were admitted to these schools. Later there were other European universities where philosophy, which was highly valued, became a component of medical education.

All the same the medicine of the Middle Ages was still in most respects just an imitation of medicine in the heyday of the ancient world. It existed only on the basis of old dogmas and there were many different sects which fought one another.

Paracelsus (1493–1541)

Paracelsus was the first physician who dared to oppose the ruling class of rigid authorities and medical dogmatism. He strongly protested against the exaggerated scientific approach to medicine, which very often prevented the right curative treatment. Paracelsus travelled very much. He went through all of Europe, from Turkey to Sweden and from France to Poland, eagerly collecting knowledge about many different ways of healing from universities, physicians and folk medicine.

The result was something completely new, and – against the expectations of other physicians – he often accomplished real miracle cures of diseases that the official medicine of his day could not heal. This was possible because he used treatments similar to ones used by Hippocrates and his disciples. Paracelsus used to say the following: 'There, where nature, somewhere in the body, produces pain many toxins have accumulated, which the organism tries to get rid of.'

Paracelsus studied the course of a disease. Only if nature could not heal a disease should the physician interfere and support the efforts of the organism to expel the toxins. Just like physicians in former times he supported the excretion of toxins by way of the skin with all possible measures. He prescribed a very personal diet for each patient, as well as remedies for the liver, remedies to induce vomiting, different herbs, laxatives and treatments, which helped the patient to perspire. He left many wonderful recipes behind.

According to him many physicians could 'only write recipes, but they could not heal anybody'. He fought against specialisation and said: 'Some specialists can do one thing and other specialists can do something else, but none of them have any real knowledge, as those who only know part of an entirety know nothing at all!'

According to him one of the main causes of disease was a poor metabolism, by means of which abnormal metabolic residues and surplus juices accumulated in the body. A sudden reflux of such substances into the interior of the body could provoke an apoplexy or other life-endangering illness. Another important cause of illness was the suppression of habitual excretions like perspiration, the respiration of the skin, menstruation and the bleeding of piles. Also too much mental as well as physical stress was, according to him, very dangerous.

Paracelsus believed in astrology and was a convinced alchemist. In his opinion all diseases were of a chemical nature and he tried to cure these with specific substances. During his entire life he tried to find the right causal remedies so that with these it would be possible to cure a disease immediately. Because of him potential remedies like lead, sulphur, iron and arsenic became known.

Although the second half of the sixteenth century was a time of many discoveries in the field of anatomy and physiology, and one would have thought that medicine would have been influenced by this in the first place, Paracelsus nevertheless remained the greatest physician of this period.

Medicine in the Seventeenth and Eighteenth Centuries

Only in the seventeenth century did the influence of exact science become stronger. It was a time in which mathematics, physics and chemistry were the dominating principles in medicine. With much enthusiasm many physicians tried to make good use of the new knowledge in their practice. However, mainly because during that period most of the traditional empirical treatments were abolished, there were frequent failures. (Bernard Aschner wrote: 'We only have to change very little to recognise the analogy to our time.')

Of course, in those times there were also several physicians who realised the dangers of such a one-sided medical approach. Santorio and his followers, such as Hufeland, pointed out how dangerous it is to prevent the natural secretions of the body. In that case caustic and irritating residues of metabolism can accumulate and pain will develop in the joints, the nerves, the muscles, the tendons, the eyes and the lungs, as well as inflammation, secretion, and deposits.

These toxins can also cause degeneration in the brain and the bone marrow. (This deserves much more notice, because even today the cause of most diseases of the nervous system still seems to be unknown!)

Sydenham (1624–1689), an English physician known as 'The English Hippocrates', encouraged the excretion of superfluous body fluids. He prescribed remedies to strengthen the stomach and according to him any one-sided diet in the long run could do more harm than good.

This time was often called the Golden Age of medicine. The Dutch physician Herman Boerhave, who was known in many countries, was a convinced Eclectic who did not believe in the value of isolated systems and did not want to submit to any dogmatic school of medicine. He tried to combine the best of all healing ways of his time.

In the eihteenth century physicians aspired to help their patients as well as they could in any possible practical way. Medicine reached a very high standard and was characterised by highly developed philosophical and practical thinking. This was supported by a many-sided knowledge of practical healing methods of the past, which is totally unknown by most physicians of our time!

Many physicians achieved successful cures, which we can only admire and from which we can learn very much. Famous physicians like Boerhave, van Swieten, Tissot and Hufeland can still show us a treasure chest filled with most effective healing methods, which have been proved many times. Doctors in those times were also of the opinion that most diseases were due to the accumulation of toxins and that these toxins always should be eliminated.

This 'humoral pathology' had the great advantage, that the physician always could use treatments which were immediately effective, because thereby harmful toxins could be excreted by way of the skin or the intestines. This kind of treatment will always be valuable. Before our time innumerable people were treated and healed by these sensible and useful treatments. Most other theories about the cause of disease in our time are just that – theoretical; they cannot be proved and prevent successful treatment.

Modern Science – Organised Obedience and Standardised Doctrines

Up until about 150 years ago medicine was more an art than a science. The physician could draw up his own recipes and on the basis of his experience he could adapt these recipes exactly to the requirements and reactions of his patients.

Around 1830 in the industrial countries a new kind of medicine developed which was based on scientific research. Medicine broke away from the old-fashioned healing methods of the past and physicians were excited about the many new therapeutic possibilities.

From the year 1850 on, modern educational establishments and research centres were built, where young scientists and physicians could be instructed. Every one of these centres had its own very definite standards which showed the exact procedures for scientific research and these centres could only afford to employ collaborators, who understood and submitted to their rules. In the course of time this trend developed more and more and the interests of each educational centre gradually became more important than the joy of discovery, knowledge, enthusiasm and tolerance.

At the beginning of the twentieth century there were vast numbers of scientists who almost without exception followed exact guidelines which were determined by the medical and pharmaceutical authorities. At the same time the chemical/pharmaceutical industry became more powerful and the major part of research was promoted and supported by that industry. Today more than ever the objective of most research is the development of new pharmaceutical products. In order to develop these products, the pharmaceutical industry employs young scientists who today, in most cases, are employed only for a fixed period. After two or three years it is decided if their achievements justify the renewal of their contract. Although at the beginning the young scientist may have the feeling that it is possible to work independently without any interference, after some time it will be realised that the results of his or her research are appreciated only when these comply with the wishes of the employer. If, because of philanthropic reasons and love of truth, this young scientist dared to question some of the expected results, pretty soon he or she would have to look for a new job.

Most scientists therefore stick to the rules, as for them this is above all a question of survival. In today's scientific community every scientist who is not financially independent has to submit to patronage by authorities or majorities. Even if a scientist because of his intelligence and his capacity for work accomplishes something exceptional, this has to be within the established borders; under these circumstances many scientists lose their creative talents.

During the development of medical drugs exact threshold limits will be determined, which in general have very little to do with their practical use. These limits – which mostly derive from animal experiments – have often been adjusted according to economic policies and only rarely for health reasons. Established limits, which should be based on practical experience gained with patients, have in these cases been decided in a totally unscientific manner.

Although in the industrial countries the pharmaceutical industry is subjected to very strict supervision, the authorities, as well as most physicians, have to depend on the scientific findings of industry. They all know very little about microbiology and therefore are only seldom able to correctly assess the real dangers of a remedy. Because today's physicians do not develop their own recipes any more, they have to make do with the prescriptions of the pharmaceutical industry and at university medical students get much information about all kinds of pharmaceutical products. The pharmaceutical industry promotes its products at university according to a very specific pattern. There are but few medical students who will take the trouble to think for themselves; most of them accept anything that is taught. They are afraid of being disqualified and therefore later in their own practice they automatically follow the path of least resistance and do what most other physicians do. However anybody who follows the crowd and does not think and act according to his or her own honest convictions becomes a stranger to themselves and denies reality and the truth.

Later on, physicians receive further training from pharmaceutical consultants, during conventions and other scientific events. As the sponsors of conventions are often pharmaceutical companies, it seems logical that most of the professional know-how given is quite specific. Afterwards all this new knowledge and new medication will be tried out on the patients.

It is an interesting observation that pharmaceutical companies, which manufacture insecticides and herbicides as well as food concentrates and additives, are all in some direct or indirect way partly responsible for the diseases which afflict so many people in today's society.

High-tech Medicine and the Decline of Our Therapeutic Abilities.

The great progress in microscopy, physiology, pathology

and pharmacology in the second half of the nineteenth century and beginning of the twentieth century was really admirable. More was constantly being learned about the human body and about many physical processes. Rudolf Virchow (1821–1902) enriched medicine with his work on leukaemia, embolism, thrombosis and many other diseases. However his most important contribution was his discovery of cellular pathology (1858), which is still fundamental for the diagnosis and treatment of disease. Thereby Virchow concluded that the cells are the most important units of life; for him disease was always the consequence of a disturbance of the normal functioning of the cells of the human body.

As a result, analytical research and the dispersal of medicine in innumerable special branches were speeded up even more. Because of this very interesting development, the former humoral pathology was totally edged out. While formerly the quantitative and qualitative composition of the body juices, especially the blood, was the most important cause of disease, now the cells were to blame for everything. People totally forgot that a healthy cell metabolism depends mostly on the condition of the nutrients, which are supplied by the blood.

Since the ousting of humoral pathology by the cellular pathology of Virchow, the healing of innumerable, especially chronic, diseases has become problematic and often impossible. In the narrow field of this one-sided vision it is no longer possible to grasp the deeper cause of the different symptoms and to choose the right treatment.

Without a general treatment of the entire body, locally applied healing methods, or tinkering around with the symptoms, are in the long run not only unsuccessful, but also dangerous. The very valuable experience of former well-known physicians has been totally ignored and in our time this has caused an immense impoverishment of healing possibilities.

During the past hundred years there have been great achievements in the field of chemistry and technical science and many dreams have come true. Without these achievements we would not know many of the comforts of modern life. Conventional medicine uses innumerable technical appliances and instruments and many physicians would feel completely lost without them.

Treating a patient originally meant that the physician had to treat the patient by using his hands. The German word 'behandeln' (to treat) has to do with the word 'hand' but an expensive practice which has been set up with many technical appliances often impresses the patient, though in most cases this has little to do with natural and effective healing. We should never forget that the mere touch of the physician during the examination of the patient already has a healing influence on the patient. This is very important. Personal contact between the physician and the patient will always be needed.

Nevertheless many modern diagnostic procedures and technical inventions can help us, as they can confirm our guesses and suspicions concerning certain diseases. Also modern technical appliances can back up some healing methods which have been known for thousands of years in a positive way, and sometimes simplify them. However it should never be forgotten that these are only auxiliary measures and that the physicians of olden times could treat and often heal diseases which now seem to be incurable without their help. Empathy, intuition and experience are far more important for a good physician than even the best technical appliances.

CHAPTER TWO

The Diagnosis

Before any treatment, whether this treatment is a traditional treatment, a homeopathic or a naturopathic treatment, there always has to be a diagnosis. Because of scientific progress it is now possible to trace even the smallest pathological changes which take place in the human body. On the basis of these findings, in combination with the case history of the patient and the medical examination, the traditionally trained physician can often make the right diagnosis. As up to the present time there are more than 60,000 different diseases known, it is not easy to make a choice and often still more laboratory or other tests are required before it is possible to give the disease in question a name.

As soon as the physician is sure of a diagnosis, he or she will be able to treat the patient according to a specific programme, which matches the illness in question. Within this programme there are several therapeutic possibilities and a choice of drugs, which is forever increasing. If one drug does not help, perhaps some other drug will do the trick and eventually most of the symptoms will disappear and the patient can be sent home, because the illness has been 'cured'.

However, modern diagnostic methods can only establish chemical and physical processes, and the changes which happen in these sectors, but life and disease involve much more! In a living organism, within fractions of seconds, hundreds and even thousands of changes take place at the same time. Although we can register more and more details, we will never be able to re-enact natural processes in a laboratory, and there are many things about the human body we do not yet know and perhaps will never know.

In modern medicine the research of details has become far too important and the number of details a physician discovers even seems to be a criterion for the capability of the physician. Many patients believe that the more details the doctor knows the better be can heal.

However, in general the opposite is true, because a physician who is obsessed by too many details can often no longer grasp the entire problem of pathological processes.

Meanwhile the patient will be impressed by all the details, as he or she, by looking at all these figures, can see for him or herself which of the available data are within an acceptable norm and which are not. When there are values – which nowadays are often found with the help of a computer – which deviate from the normal standard, the physician will make a choice of the available therapeutic solutions to the problem. If the physician happens to be a good chemist and technician, he will be able to judge the laboratory values exactly. In that case he will know what to do and the patient will be treated according to the rules.

One would think that with so much knowledge most diseases would be cured without any problems. Unfortunately this is not so. Despite spectacular diagnostic findings and enormous financial investment, people in the past hundred years have not become any healthier, but on the contrary, much more ill. How is that possible? It is because all these laboratory and other tests usually have little to do with the real causes of the disease. Most of these symptoms only indicate the changes which take place in the organism when, because of too many toxins and other negative influences, the natural equilibrium in the body has been lost. Even after most of these values have been corrected – often by dangerous means – the disease itself has not disappeared.

If medicine would not interfere, many of these abnormal diagnostic findings after some time would generally change again all by themselves; in a living organism nothing will stay the same for any length of time. However if one tries to suppress these symptoms with unnatural measures, it is like disconnecting the fire alarm, while nothing is being done about the fire itself. Unfortunately the entire construction of officially recognised medicine is based on this serious error.

I do not condemn modern medicine and its diagnostic methods, but I do condemn the way in which diagnostic findings are interpreted and exploited to the disadvantage of the patients, although most physicians do not even realise this.

Modern medicine is and always will be a medicine exclusively for emergencies and in this respect it really can be admired.

The Right Kind of Diagnosis

Although the above-mentioned diagnostics have nothing to do with the cause of the disease, all the same they can   -

be used as control values. To be precise, if by natural means the health of the patient has improved his diagnostic values also will have changed for the better.

An intelligent and talented practitioner or healer always wants to know the original cause of the illness, which usually lies hidden under many layers of secondary symptoms. Without this knowledge it is not possible to treat the patient in the right way. Because of this, the practitioner should be informed of all details concerning the lifestyle and nutritional habits of his patients, and he should take all the complaints of his patients seriously, even if these, according to other physicians, have been only imaginary.

Although in our time most practitioners have no time for a thorough examination of the patient it would still be very important to examine the abdomen of the patient with great care, like the Mayr doctors are taught to do. This is extremely important, as at least 80 per cent of all the diseases of modern society stem from problems in the intestinal tract. Physicians of former times could detect the origin of a disease just by looking at the posture of the body and many other signs.

The Art of Semiotics

Semiotics, the art of detecting the symptoms, is as old as mankind itself. Many physicians of olden times had a complete command of this kind of diagnosis. By simply observing the patient they could detect many health problems, whereas today's medical students do not know anything, or only very little, about the great advantages this knowledge can bring.

Many of them think that semiotics belongs to another

era and they cannot imagine a situation without diagnostic appliances and laboratory tests. They have never learned to really observe their patients. As a result of technical development, the information obtained by the naked eye usually gets lost.

The artist in the physician will be attracted by semiotics, which uses feelings like instinct, intuition, the talent of observation and the ability to understand biological connections. Physicians of the old school looked at the tongue, the hands and the nails, as well as at the condition and the colour of the skin and many other features of the patient. Elderly relatives or friends will perhaps remember a time when doctors would ask patients to show their tongue.

Diagnosis and Treatment Through Reflex Centres

Even in olden times, doctors knew the value of reflex centres. Such centres are not only found on the feet. They can be found all over the body and they all follow complicated nerve tracts, which are connected with nerve centres in the brain.

All body parts and organs are accessible via corresponding reflex points at different places under the skin. Not only is it possible to treat an organ or body part by rubbing or pressing the corresponding reflex zone, it is also possible to make a diagnosis the same way. When a reflex zone really hurts, this is always a sign that there is something wrong with the corresponding organs or body parts.

If the blood circulation of a certain organ is impaired because of the accumulation of toxins, this is also noticeable in the corresponding reflex centres. In that case specific areas on the back, for example, often near the spine, will be painful or maybe swollen or on the contrary these areas will lie a little deeper under the skin and form a dent. A doctor trained in biological diagnosis will always inspect the back and other parts of the body in order to find such swellings or dents. In reflex centres which correspond with the diseased organs one finds accumulations of toxins, lymphatic fluid or fat, although on a much smaller scale than in the organ itself. These toxins have sometimes been accumulating there for years until the corresponding reflex zone becomes painful.

All such abnormalities of the skin are very important, because by using special poultices or blistering paper the physician has the opportunity to eliminate toxins, right away and on the spot. Superficial health problems and also diseases deep in the body can be treated like this. In Asian and Arabic medicine such effective healing methods were already being used thousands of years ago. However, as such treatments take much time and do not make much money, official medicine was never really interested in them. Such things are not taught at university; only the so-called empirical medicine in Germany has tried to awaken interest in these methods. Meanwhile they are a real blessing for naturopaths and their patients.

A REGULAR BOWEL FUNCTION IS EXTREMELY IMPORTANT

The physician should always ask his patients about the functioning of their bowels. Many people are still under the impression that digestive disorders have little or nothing to do with their state of health. However, irregular bowel movements can cause severe blockages and dangerous diseases, not only of the intestines but of the entire organism. Nowadays 90 per cent of the inhabitants of the industrial countries suffer from mild or serious gastric irregularities.

THE TEETH
A further important indication of the state of health is the condition of the teeth. According to Dr Bircher-Benner, caries are a reliable sign of serious general health problems caused by wrong nutrition. Also diseases of the gums and periodontosis (loose teeth) are such signs. Gold crowns, bridges and so on are signs of former malnutrition. (See *10 Golden Rules for Good Health*) Even one carious tooth indicates that there is something wrong with the metabolism. Sweets not only damage teeth from the outside, but as any kind of industrially produced sugar causes a lack of vital substances, the teeth and the jawbones become weaker and the composition of the saliva changes.

DISEASE-PROVOKING LIVING HABITS
Are Waerland, the well-known Swedish nutritional scientist, said: 'Diseases develop because of mistakes in nutritional and living habits; when you remove the mistakes the diseases disappear by themselves.' Bircher-Benner said that diseases are always caused by a disorder in the person's lifestyle and that such disorders often develop during childhood. By disorder, he meant all behaviour that offends against the natural laws of life. Only if the physician can find out about all the different aspects of disorder in the life of his patient will he or she be able to help. 'Only in this way,' said Bircher-Benner 'will it be possible to build a bridge from the diagnosis to the therapy', and modern medicine has lost the blueprints of such a bridge.

Since the time of Bircher-Benner the disorders in people's lives have increased tremendously, mainly in the industrialised countries, and at the same time the diseases which are the theme of this book have increased in a frightening way. Diseases which a hundred years ago were hardly known now threaten the health of millions of people. Only a physician who is able to make the right diagnosis will be able to build this bridge, which will make it possible to give patients real help.

The search for the real causes behind all the different symptoms is extremely important. As Professor Zabel said: 'Behind a large number of diseases there are only a few causes. To reveal these causes and to eliminate them, instead of blundering about the symptoms, is the most important task of today's physician.'

CHAPTER THREE

The Right Treatment
of Modern Diseases

Guidelines for Treatment

To successfully treat rheumatic diseases, allergies and other diseases, the most important causes of such diseases should be first of all be eliminated and these always include wrong eating habits, an unhealthy lifestyle, lack of exercise and any mental problems of the person in question.

The following guidelines should be observed.

1. It is essential that no further toxins get into the body.
2. A change of diet should be done step by step and never be hurried.
3. The patient should always enjoy his food and fasting, some mono diet or a cure with cereal jelly can be of great help.
4. In the case of mental disease, not only the mind but also the body should be treated and vice versa. The patient should be given the opportunity to speak about his or her problems.
5. Before starting a treatment the physician always

should find out if the excretory organs are healthy and if they function correctly. If not, they should be treated in the first place.

6. The physician should clean the organism at all levels, step by step, while observing the reactions of the patient.

7. Only then, when the cleaning process is finished, will the physician begin to build up the defence system of the body, with the help of natural therapies and remedies. To treat the patient in any other way would be wrong and a waste of valuable energy.

The Responsibility of the Patient

It is not the doctor, the chemist, the health insurance company, the pharmaceutical industry or the government that should be responsible for our health. We ourselves should take care of our health and the health of our family and we ought to do all we can in order to prevent serious illness.

Until quite recently, patients thought they were free of any personal responsibility concerning their health. Apparently it was not their fault that they fell ill, and they were not expected to recover on their own. This suited most patients very well. They gladly accepted treatment from their physicians. After all, nobody wants to be involved in something he or she cannot understand. Therefore we have physicians and nurses. If anything happens medical staff are supposed to help us.

However, lately things have changed somewhat. In the industrial countries the public have become aware that something is very wrong indeed. If a patient blindly follows medical advice it can happen that the disease, instead of getting better, often gets worse and sometimes even becomes incurable. Intelligent patients have woken up and realised that they are fully entitled to know more about their illness and about the functioning of their body. They want to know more about the medication they are given and, above all, about why they became ill.

This, however, seems to be the biggest problem of all, as on this subject there is no real and honest information available, not even for physicians or medical students! Nobody seems to know why we become ill and according to statistics, doctors are almost at the top of the list for most diseases, like those of the liver, the kidneys and the lungs, as well as diabetes and cardiovascular diseases. If doctors knew the causes of illness they would not become ill.

Subconsciously most patients know more or less why they are ill. By using their brains as they should be used, physicians as well as their patients would be able to understand the most important causes of disease. They would change their eating and living habits and take on responsibility for their own health.

Positive Healing Reactions

In medicine there are two kinds of so-called 'side effects'. Side effects of remedies which most physicians prescribe in order to suppress symptoms are sometimes more dangerous than the illness itself. Natural remedies can also have side effects. However these side effects are on the contrary 'positive healing reactions' which are beneficial for our health. When reading the chapter about the different stages of illness (Dr Reckeweg) you will know that the more often the symptoms are suppressed, the more the health of the person in question deteriorates. Step by step the disease comes into the next stage until the patient will be chronically and sometimes incurably ill.

Not only Dr Reckeweg but all open-minded physicians and good naturopaths know that serious illness can only be cured when the patient experiences again all the different stages of illness (this time in reverse order). In this way all the different stages of disease, which constantly were suppressed, have at last the opportunity to heal. Again the patient will relive all the different diseases, beginning with the disease from which he is suffering at the present time and ending with simple health problems like the common cold and step by step his or her health will improve. All the intensive cleaning procedures have to start at the top layer and work down to the bottom. However this time the duration of all these diseases will be very short and the symptoms that thereby occur are positive healing reactions.

The physician or therapist will always observe all healing reactions very carefully and he will see to it that the patient has enough strength to be able to cope with the next reaction. This needs much knowledge, understanding and empathy. Such positive healing reactions, which are absolutely necessary, can be set off on purpose by different natural therapies and remedies mentioned in this book. Only in this way very seriously ill patients might improve or in some cases even be completely cured.

Prevention and Treatment of Disease

It is extremely important that anybody who notices there is something wrong with his or her health does something about it. The following rules should be followed:

1. Eat simple, natural and healthy food and never too much.
2. Clean the intestines and sanitise the intestinal flora.
3. Be sure to have a regular bowel movement.
4. Stimulants like coffee, tobacco, alcohol, drugs and so on are forbidden.
5. Take plenty of exercise in the fresh air.
6. It is important to perspire each day.
7. It is important to stimulate the mind.
8. If possible, take no more chemical medication.
9. In the case of high blood pressure take no medication, but begin a course of regular bloodletting administered by a physician experienced in this art.
10. Plenty of sleep, regular relaxation and minimal stress are essential.
11. Natural or homeopathic medicaments to improve the brain function should be used, for example ginkgo biloba.

CHAPTER FOUR

Our Excretory Organs

Our most important excretory organs are the intestines, the liver, the kidneys (and the bladder), the lungs and the skin. All toxins are excreted via the blood, the lymph and other body fluids, as well as via the gases which come from the lungs. The body protects itself permanently through self-cleaning measures. What we call disease is simply the consequence of the body's efforts to excrete harmful substances which endanger our health. We know that any man-made machine can only deal with a certain amount of work for a certain period of time. The same happens with the different excretory organs of the human body.

Most health problems are due to the accumulation of toxic matter. Because of this it is highly important to first clean the organism via the excretory organs and in other ways before trying to cure a disease. Only when because of over-exertion, weakness or for other reasons these important and natural excretory processes do not function well, should the physician interfere and carefully support the healing efforts of the organism in the best way possible. However, while doing this he or she should never overtax any single excretory organ with a tiring treatment. The best thing is to activate the different excretory organs one after the other and at the same time support the liver and the gall bladder with natural remedies.

The Intestines

Most diseases of our time have their roots in our intestinal tract and therefore it is logical to start all cleaning measures there. Although hardly anybody realises this, the intestines of most elderly, and also of a great number of younger people, have lost their original shape and are deformed. As a result many important functions of the intestines are impaired. Hard, dried-up residues of excrement may remain for a long time, sometimes for years, in the intestinal loops and stick to the intestinal wall. This situation has to be corrected in the first place, as without cleaning the intestines it is not possible to heal any disease.

There are several ways in which this cleaning may be done. Every morning an enema should be administered, using two litres of warm water or herbal tea, so that by and by most old residues can be dissolved. If the problem is more serious, the physician may prescribe several treatments of 'colon hydrotherapy', whereby the intestines will be washed out with about 40 litres of water, sometimes with the addition of oxygen.

This therapy is usually done twice a week for about four to six weeks; more often is not advisable, as the intestines would dry out too much. During this therapy it will be good, once in a while, to inject a little natural oil into the anus with a syringe (but without the needle!). This treatment should always be combined with the sanitation of the intestinal flora, by taking special enzymes and homeopathic remedies.

As mental health is closely connected with the health of the intestines, for many years physicians have successfully treated mentally ill or depressive patients with colon hydrotherapy. In cases of mood swings or extreme nervousness it would be advisable to try this.

THE PROBLEM OF CONSTIPATION

Almost all refined and industrially changed food causes constipation. When people eat too much of this kind of food, the little filters in the intestinal wall get clogged up and as a consequence fewer nutrients can pass into the blood. In this way, after some time the organism will become undernourished. When the intestines have been cleaned and the exchange of nutrients is normal again people blossom. When no more toxins get into the organism it at last has the chance to become healthy.

Strong laxatives should be used only in an emergency. Laxatives may help momentarily, but they will not resolve the problem and in the long run they only make things worse. They weaken the muscles of the intestinal wall and the stool can no longer be excreted in a natural way. When taking laxatives sometimes only part of the contents of the intestines will be excreted and often old and hard crusts stay where they are for days, months or even for years.

Castor oil or different herbal mixtures can also help to clean the intestines, but even these can be too strong for sensitive people. A physician who has learned about natural treatments will always choose the therapies and remedies which will suit his or her patient best.

In past times many natural laxatives were known. Although some physicians still prescribe plant jellies, which of course are less harmful then most modern drugs, unfortunately innumerable recipes have been lost or forgotten. Linseed is highly recommended, as it contains much mucous. Here is the recipe: a few soup-spoons of linseed should be soaked in some water overnight and a small amount of this can be added to drinks, soup or broth several times a day. Usually the stool will soon become normal. Dried figs, apricots or plums soaked overnight are also good laxatives.

Drinking a glass of warm water early in the morning or, better still, an enema early in the morning stimulates the stool. This is done with a so-called 'rubber pear' which can be bought in a pharmacy, or with an enema syringe. Small cold-water enemas given at night will help to soften the stool while the patient is sleeping.

GASTRITIS AND SIMILAR PROBLEMS
If the problems are not yet severe it would be advisable to prevent further damage. For quite some time one should not eat anything raw – no raw vegetables, salads or fruits – and substitute these with steamed vegetables, vegetable soup, boiled cereals, cereal jelly, Swedish knackebrot, fresh goat's cheese with herbs, oats or barley soup.

If the patient has the opportunity to go to a clinic that specialises in intestinal cleaning, a Mayr cure can be recommended. This cure consists of a very simple diet, whereby the intestines have a chance to recuperate. In Mayr clinics special massages of the abdomen, physiotherapy and hydrotherapy are used. A similar diet could be followed at home however there are not many people who really have the willpower to do this in the right way.

It is easier to do a cereal jelly cure, for example (see chapter six), by which many gastric problems and even some serious diseases can be cured. For still better results, cleaning of the intestines can be supported by fasting or by following a very simple diet and by drinking special herbal teas.

FASTING IN THE RIGHT WAY

The well-known physician Herbert Shelton wrote a book called *Fasting Can Save Your Life* and indeed this is true. Unfortunately, there are many people who are afraid to fast. They believe that fasting is something unnatural and they also believe that one can starve to death while fasting, as the human body always needs food. These people do not know that on the contrary fasting is very natural. Not only human beings but also animals and even plants fast once in a while.

However, it is understandable that some people do not dare to fast, because we know that, after a hunger-strike, participants sometimes die. These people die because they fast in a dangerous way without enough knowledge about what really happens in our body when we are fasting. Any healthy person can fast for four weeks, or even longer, without any danger. Fasting as such is not difficult at all, but one should know exactly how to behave when the time of fasting is over. It is unbelievable that some otherwise intelligent people go on a fast without being well informed about the subject.

When a person goes on a fast he or she only needs much willpower for the first day or two. On the second or third day he or she may not feel well, as many changes will then be taking place in the body and its digestive processes will be changing. On this day, the person in question should stay in bed reading or listening to some music for distraction.

After the organism has adapted to the new situation,

most people feel very good during the rest of the fast, and generally they do not feel hungry at all; they often feel rather euphoric and happy.

Fasting means a real housecleaning for the organism. Once in a while during a fast it can happen that too many toxins are dissolved at one time and enter into the bloodstream. When this happens, the excretory organs often become overtaxed. Then the person in question does not feel well until the problem has been solved. Such healing reactions are completely normal during the process of elimination. After such a reaction, which usually only lasts a few hours, the health of the patient will improve greatly and the effort will have been worthwhile!

When terminating a fast one should not start eating normally right away as this could be life-threatening. The reason for this is that during the fast the organism produces fewer and fewer digestive juices because they are not needed. If after a longer fast someone eats, for example, a cheese sandwich, there are no digestive juices whatever available for the digestion of the cheese, the butter and the bread. Such digestive juices have to be produced again by the organism and this cannot be done immediately. The food will lie in the body like a lead weight and act like a poison. No wonder that because of such stupid behaviour a faster may even die!

To end a fast means starting to eat again very slowly, step by step. This is far more difficult than the actual fasting itself. It is not easy to restrain oneself when starting to eat again, for from that moment on one starts to feel hungry once more and that feeling will have disappeared during the fast. Now much willpower is needed.

As a rule just as much time is needed before starting to

eat normally again as the time that has passed during the fast. So if one fasts for two weeks, two weeks will be needed before it is possible to eat normally again. It is advisable to take, for example, a glass of carrot juice mixed with water and to drink this very slowly sip by sip three to five times on the first day. In this way the organism may begin to produce the required digestive juices.

On the second day it is possible to take the juice without water. In between, when thirsty, one can, of course, drink all the water one likes. Start with some grated carrots or apples on the third day. Always eat very slowly and chew the food for a very long time. After about a week it will be possible to start eating some boiled vegetables and potatoes and from that time on it is advisable to eat no more than three times a day in order to give the digestive organs plenty of rest between meals. Mainly because of acidity reactions, fruit is permitted only much later.

During the first two or three weeks after the fast only very small portions should be eaten and only one or two kinds of food at each meal, and the food should be eaten very slowly, so that the food is mixed with plenty of saliva. For a long time after the fast, no, or only very little, animal protein should be eaten. If one starts eating normally too soon, perhaps because one is impatient, or if one eats the wrong kind of food or eats too fast, former health problems may return. Everybody is able to fast, but when the fast is over everyone should know what to do and have enough intelligence and willpower to start eating again in the right way.

There are many good books about fasting. Before you start on a fast, please read as much as possible on the subject. Everyone has their own tastes and different eating habits and when the fast is over you will be able to create your own health diet. If you want help, look for a physician who is knowledgeable on the subject and has plenty of experience.

The Liver

The liver is a very important excretory organ, which also detoxifies many harmful substances. We have to make sure that our liver always remains healthy and is able to carry out its 50 or even more tasks in an optimum way.

It is largely in the liver that toxic substances which might damage the cells are rendered harmless. Waste products from worn-out cell proteins are broken down and the liver transforms toxins into harmless substances, which by way of the kidneys are excreted through the urine. Furthermore, the liver produces gall fluids and with these fluids toxic substances can be excreted into the small intestine via the bile ducts.

In the liver there are numerous tiny filters which rid the blood of all kinds of toxins and germs. The liver and the gall bladder empty their residues into different channels, which finally end up in the bowels from where these residues are excreted. However, sometimes the liver has to cope with too many toxins at one time and it can also happen that not enough bile may be produced. This is noticeable when we cannot digest fats, when we suffer from gastric problems, from stomach-ache or from pain in the upper part of the abdomen after a meal. In that case a special liver diet with very little or no fat, with the exception of some cold-pressed oil and special herbal teas, may help.

Pain in the right side, in the middle of the body, may

be due to liver trouble. When the person in question also suffers from wind and has a bloated feeling there may be a build-up of toxins in the liver. If this pain occurs mainly under or above the liver, the colour of the stool is too light and cholesterol is too high, this is also a sign of such a build-up of toxins. Whey diluted with some water is an excellent remedy. Never use vinegar, as this is very dangerous for the liver. For the purification of the liver, artichokes, radishes, dandelions, olive oil and bitter teas are very helpful.

There are many more natural remedies and therapies which support the work of the liver. Warm humid compresses, clay compresses, or compresses prepared with the oil of St John's Wort can be applied on the liver after meals. Using horse chestnut or horsetail as a compress will bring great relief. These compresses can stay on all night.

Although in general fat is bad for the liver, it is completely wrong to eat no fat at all, as the liver needs some unsaturated oil. However, this oil should never be heated – no fried potatoes, chips or any fried food! As soon as fat or even butter is heated, it becomes saturated and saturated fats are extremely bad for the liver. Some cold-pressed virgin oil has exactly the opposite effect; it supports the healing of the liver. The label 'virgin' means that the oil comes from the first pressing of the oil from olives or sunflower seeds, or other seeds, nuts or plants.

Liver patients always need some protein, but it is important to know what kind of protein. For example, eggs in any form are bad for the liver; it is certainly less harmful for the patient to eat some lean meat once in a while. As vegetables or cereals usually do not contain much protein, it would be advisable to eat each day a little quark, cottage cheese or natural yoghurt without sugar or chemical additives from the healthfood store. Milk is forbidden, because in every glass of milk there is a surplus of acids and for the same reason so are all citrus fruits, and any other fruits or vegetables which contain too much acid. For instance cooked fruit and incorrectly cooked vegetables, are bad for the liver.

Strong spices are dangerous for the liver, but food can be made very appetising by using different fresh herbs. Whey, carrot juice, the juice of raw potatoes and, above all, ground-up sesame seeds, flax seeds and their oils are excellent for the liver.

Liver remedies are: solidago (goldenrod), podophyllum D4-D6, chelidonium D4 and taraxacum (dandelion). The patient also needs B-complex vitamins and vitamins A and E.

The Kidneys

If important excretory organs of the body degenerate and do not function well any more, this can have disastrous consequences. Healthy blood and plenty of oxygen are needed for the optimal functioning of the kidneys. The kidneys need much more oxygen than the liver as far more blood circulates through the kidneys than the other organs. Every 24 hours, 1,440 litres of blood pass through the kidneys. This blood contains many toxins, which are filtered there. The more blood flows through the kidneys, the better. In the case of low blood pressure, less blood than normal flows through the kidneys. When the weather is warm the kidneys function better than when it is cold. No other organ, with the exception of the heart and the liver, will suffer so much when we have wrong nutritional habits and eat processed food as our kidneys. Highly concentrated products especially, like sugar and white flour, do a lot of harm.

Most kidney diseases are the consequence of too much acidity. This happens when the person in question eats too much refined food and salt or drinks too much coffee, alcohol or cold drinks other than water. About 80 per cent of our modern food is far too acidic; in the time of our grandparents, acidic food constituted no more than about 20 per cent of a normal diet.

The blood of people who do not live healthily contains many toxins, which have to be filtered out by their kidneys. These toxins are then diluted in water and excreted in the urine, so drinking plenty of water is very important. Alcoholic drinks, coffee, tea and soft drinks have the opposite effect; those drinks dry the body out.

The kidneys are not designed to process chemical or synthetic substances (like some drugs or food additives); such substances block or damage the small filters of the kidneys. In this way blockages and/or inflammations of the kidneys can occur. Sometimes because of cold weather and even because of emotional problems, the cleaning procedures of the kidney filters can also become blocked. The patient who has kidney trouble usually feels weak and tired; many of these patients suffer from oedemas, or swellings of a dropsical nature, because of water retention. Often their urine becomes cloudy and dirty or sometimes the colour is reddish brown and the quantity can also be too little. Usually the blood pressure is normal, but when the disease is serious this can be very high.

If there are aches and pains in the area of the kidneys when the person in question is in a reclining position or when getting up, generally there is something wrong with the kidneys. In order to know if you are dealing with a weakness or a disease of the kidneys, you should measure the intake of liquids over a period of 24 hours, as well as the quantity of urine during that period. In this way it is possible to know if you pass enough urine. It is best to do this test over three successive days.

Another test, and remedy at the same time, is to follow the diet of Dr Kousa or the wheat-jelly cure for four days. If one has to urinate very much during that time, it is a sure sign that there has been an accumulation of too many liquids in the kidneys.

The functions of all the inner organs link up very closely and if the kidneys are no longer able to eliminate enough toxins, other organs will take over part of the work. In this case different secondary symptoms may develop. In the mornings the person in question may get headaches or migraine. They may suffer from ringing in the ears, dizziness, puffy eyelids, a rapid heartbeat, anxiety, skin rashes and changes of pigmentation, especially at folds of skin. There can be a burning sensation in the anus, varicose ulcers, gout, high blood pressure and so on. If the skin takes over some of the work, there can be different kinds of skin diseases, like psoriasis or neurodermatitis. Many of these symptoms improve as soon as the kidneys are treated in the right way with natural methods.

SIDE EFFECTS
However, if such secondary symptoms are treated with strong medication, the excretion of toxins by way of the skin is often made impossible. As a consequence of such wrong treatment serious kidney diseases can occur. Sometimes the lungs will take over part of this difficult task and then the person in question after some time will start suffering from bronchitis or become asthmatic.

Some pharmaceutical remedies, like diuretics, which are prescribed in the case of a poor urine excretion, may have serious side effects. A typical side effect of this kind of remedy is a loss of salt and there is a danger of thrombosis because of blood coagulation; also the acid content of the blood increases (gout). The blood sugar level becomes higher (diabetes), and because of a decrease of the blood pressure, people feel dizzy, become constipated and often become very confused.

KIDNEY STONES
Kidney stones can be extremely painful. They are usually caused by a diet containing too much protein and acid-producing food and a lack of vitamins and exercise. They cause chronic constipation and chronic cold feet. Caffeine, black tea, cacao and alcohol are very bad for the kidneys. Often there is an inherited weakness of the kidneys. Kidney stones sometimes cause a great sensitivity in the groin. Gall stone attacks are very painful, but this pain generally radiates to the right shoulder.

RECOMMENDED TREATMENTS FOR KIDNEY TROUBLE
In order to prevent serious kidney diseases or to treat these, it is very important to clean the kidneys once in a while, through the skin. A physician who knows about the treatments of Hippocrates will be able to find abnormal sensitive places on the skin. In the case of kidney diseases or other diseased organs, there will be either elevated or indented areas on the patient's back. There the physician will do some cupping so that the toxins are freed and can be excreted from the body. Cantharid plasters can also work wonders, but it is very important to remember that these plasters should never

be used near the kidneys, as they may dry the kidneys out. To use these plasters there could be dangerous.

Hip-baths whereby the temperature of the water gradually increases, followed by wet packs, are excellent for kidney problems. When it is impossible for the patient to urinate, often a very warm hip-bath with special herbal decoctions can be successful. At the same time the patient should have an enema twice a day, so that the intestines are completely cleaned. The healthy intestines can take over much of the work and the kidneys will not be overtaxed any longer.

Regular enemas, induced perspiration, sunbathing (sensibly) and bloodletting are recommended. A few spoonfuls of olive oil every day and massages of the abdomen ensure a regular stool.

The feet of the patient should always be kept warm; when the feet are cold the best way to improve the circulation is through so-called 'Schiele baths', a foot-bath in which the temperature of the water is gradually increased. Drying the feet with a rough towel is also good for the circulation. If the patient has a temperature or there is blood or protein in the urine, bed-rest is necessary. Brushing the body all over and washing briskly with cold water is excellent.

In the case of kidney problems a change of diet is always recommended and above all the patient should eat very little protein, especially animal protein, which can do a lot of harm. A healthy and simple diet is the best insurance against kidney diseases. As long as one has kidney problems this advice should always be followed. A fruit diet including diluted fruit juices can be good for a kidney patient. However one should never eat raw fruits and vegetables when suffering from gastric problems or flatulence. Only when these problems have been overcome can the person in question slowly begin to try to start eating some raw vegetables.

Good diuretic and anti-inflammatory remedies are:

> Vegetables: corn (maize), onions, cress, leeks, cabbage, fennel, celery, parsley and green beans. Fruit: apples, cherries, plums, blackcurrants. Curative herbs: lime blossom, dandelion, heather, beech and birch leaves, wheat grass, nettle, hawthorn, elderberry and chamomile. Rubia is an excellent remedy in the case of kidney attacks.

When therapeutic injections (procaine) are given in certain acupuncture points it is amazing how quickly the pain of a kidney attack disappears. These procaine injections are often mixed with homeopathic substances, which help fight cramps.

The Lungs

The lungs are provided with excellent defence mechanisms. Many waste products from the body are transported there by way of the blood. The lungs supply oxygen and dispose of carbon dioxide. In the lung alveoli, the tiny air sacs in the lungs, waste products are converted into gases so that they can be exhaled. The respiratory organs are the exit for all waste products in the form of gas.

Though it is always extremely important to remember that all functions in the body are closely related, most physicians are hardly taught about such things. Therefore, in the case of a lung disease, a lung specialist will prescribe mainly remedies and treatments that are specific to the lungs. However, chemical drugs do no more than suppress the symptoms and should be used only in emergencies. There are natural remedies and herbs that may really help.

Many lung diseases are caused in a direct way, by toxins that have been inhaled by way of the nose or the mouth, and we all know that smoking and the inhaling of strong chemicals is poisonous for our lungs. But what about people who do not smoke or are not exposed to certain chemicals during their work? In that case the lung disease has probably originated elsewhere in the body. The mucous membrane of the respiratory tract is closely connected with the skin and the mucous membranes of the stomach, the intestines and the kidneys. When the food is unhealthy and the kidneys are unable to excrete sufficient toxins, usually the skin is the first organ that takes over the work of the kidneys. If the patient is not able to perspire enough and the pores of his skin have been clogged up for some reason, few toxins can leave the organism in that way. When the kidneys as well as the skin cannot excrete enough toxins, the rest of the work has to be done by the intestines. However, often because of chronic constipation or gastric problems, it can happen that the intestines also cannot excrete enough waste products.

If all the other organs are already overworked most 'of the waste products will be sent to the lungs, which function as a kind of emergency exit. In that case the excretive function of the lungs will be terribly overtaxed and often this is the cause of lung diseases.

Normally solid substances cannot get through the walls of the lung alveoli, but in our time more and more toxic chemicals and synthetic substances irritate the mucous membranes of the lung alveoli and injure them.

In the long run these alveoli become blocked up or porous. If the latter happens, foreign matter can enter the lungs and as a consequence the accumulation of putrefactive substances in the lungs will increase and harmful germs will also multiply rapidly.

Often, in combination with other negative factors like colds and flu, weakness, dampness, cold weather and the inhaling of smoke, dust or germs, diseases of the respiratory tract can occur.

Smoking

As we all know smoking and passive smoking are amongst the most dangerous causes of disease. At the time of writing 42 different kinds of toxins are known to be present in tobacco. Often smokers suffer from a chronic cough or from bronchitis. After smoking for many years, the lung alveoli begin to look like the carbonised leaves of a tree. Lung cancer is very dangerous and is usually caused by smoking. Most smokers cannot get rid of their addiction, though sometimes hypnosis or ear acupuncture may help.

The diet should be very simple without any industrially prepared foods. As milk produces mucous, milk and all milk products are strictly forbidden. Watch out for hidden milk (for example in bread). Many lung patients are allergic to certain foods, like citrus fruits, wheat, tomatoes etc. A 'dry diet', including dry bread and prunes and so on, can be very helpful. Such a diet loosens up the mucous and cleans the lymphatic system.

Constipation can poison the organism from the inside and because of this the patient should take an enema two or three times a day. An intestinal bath once in a while can give much relief to a lung patient. In order to take some of the strain off the lungs, the other excretive organs, especially the intestines should be treated so that they can take over some of the work, and this is something that lung specialists should learn about. Hydrotherapy, sunbathing and massage of the inner nasal passages will help. In the past, to treat lung diseases mustard poultices would be placed on the breast and kept there until there was a burning sensation. Cupping, inhalations of herbal extracts, poultices with quark (fresh white cheese) or essential oils, neural therapy and plenty of fresh air have all helped lung patients for thousands of years.

Lung patients should do some regular exercise, but this should never be overdone. When a patient suffers from flatulence or other gastric problems they should not eat raw food until their intestinal problems have been cured. People suffering from lung diseases need much organic calcium. There are very good homeopathic remedies, like calcium phosphoricum D4, D6 or D12, or Urticalcin.

It is possible to make organic calcium at home from two or more eggs. These should come from chickens raised in a natural way. These eggs should be put into the juice of four lemons and turned every second day. After a week the eggs can be thrown away and the lemon juice can be taken regularly. This lemon juice with calcium can always be prepared anew.

The Skin

A healthy skin should be soft, warm and supplied with plenty of blood. Unfortunately there are more and more people who have an unhealthy skin. Fat cells and waste products prevent respiration and blood circulation in the upper layers of the skin. The skin in this case is cold and rough or fat and shiny, and with a skin like that it is very difficult to perspire. Later there will be more and more dead cells and as the skin becomes thicker, corns, warts and even psoriasis may develop.

A healthy skin breathes, and through this about 500 to 700 grams of gaseous toxins are excreted every day. You have probably seen horses which, when the weather is cold, look as if steam is coming out of their bodies. The same happens to people, but one cannot see it. About one-third of all toxins are eliminated daily through the skin and it can have serious consequences for our health if this form of detoxification does not function properly.

TREATMENTS FOR SKIN PROBLEMS

Anyone whose skin does not function properly should do everything possible to improve the blood circulation. To achieve this all methods of hydrotherapy, massages, rubbing, brushing of the skin and reflexology are very effective. Exercise is excellent for the skin, for instance walking, running and swimming, as is plenty of fresh air. Last but not least, a healthy diet is extremely important for the health and the appearance of the skin.

As an excretory organ our skin is at least as important as our kidneys. The skin is our biggest excretive organ, containing about three million cells. For cleaning purposes each centimetre of skin contains 12–15 sebaceous glands and 90–120 sweat glands. Excretion through the skin has been promoted since primeval times. Primitive people treated pain by scratching, rubbing and sucking. The Greeks and other people of ancient times used cupping in order to draw harmful substances from deep in the body to the surface of the skin. The Romans used certain liquids which made the skin sore and sensitive, whereby the tiny lymph channels opened up and toxins could be discharged. Through cupping and similar treatments many degenerative diseases, for example of the joints, could be treated and even sometimes be cured. In the Middle Ages substances called postulants and vesicants were used. These caused rashes and blisters. When these ripened and opened up small sores were left, from which fluid would leak. Often at the same time pain and other symptoms disappeared, even such pain as originated deep in the body. Later, Paracelsus also used such poultices or liquids. In this way and by making artificial ulcers, he cured arthritis, eye diseases and even epilepsy. Hufeland also treated his patients in this way. He said: 'The art of artificial ulcers is great. They can even break down the worst ankylosis (hardening of the joints)'. When treating a patient using artificial ulcers physicians would burn little holes into the skin (cauterisation) and then put a tiny stone into the hole. After some days the small wound would start festering and an artificial ulcer appear. Through these ulcers many health problems were cured and it was possible to treat successfully severe pain, inflammation, neuritis, neuralgia, sciatica, gout and even some mental diseases.

Since ancient times people have promoted the excretion of harmful toxins through the skin by using tattoos or moxibustion, whereby the skin is lightly burned, as well as through the methods mentioned above. Very early it was discovered that the bites from ants and other insects, as well as nettle stings, had a good influence on health. We still know the positive effect of mustard compounds and mustard paper and a footbath with mustard is one of the best treatments when one has to divert the flow of lymphatic fluids. In folk medicine different resins, essential oils, paraffin and petrol have been used to provoke skin irritations. Petrol compresses are helpful in cases of lumbago, sciatica, sprains and diseases of the joints.

Which treatment is best for the patient depends on many different factors, for example the constitution, the gender, the pigmentation of the skin, previous diseases, the race, environmental influences, the defence mechanisms and the responsiveness of the person in question. Apart from all kinds of hydro-therapeutic treatments, which will be described later, important excretory methods in the treatment of many diseases are perspiration, cupping, the Baunscheidt treatment and, above all, cantharidal plasters. All of these methods will shortly be described in full. Deep down in the body such treatments have a far-reaching influence as through them harmful substances are brought up to the surface, so that they can be excreted. With the suppression of symptoms the opposite will be achieved.

DIET AND SKIN TROUBLE

A healthy and simple diet should contain no, or only very little, animal products. Ham (and any other meat from the pig) and eggs are strictly forbidden! No sweets, pastry, refined foods, soft drinks or any junk food should be permitted. No fried foods, cheese, milk or milk products, with the exception of a little quark now and then. People who have skin trouble need much calcium from vegetables and grains. A natural calcium product like Urticalcin is also excellent, as well as the homemade calcium remedy described above.

SKIN CARE

While washing, especially when using soap, natural oil is removed from the skin and therefore it is advisable to apply some good oil, like that of St John's Wort, on the skin after washing. It is even better to mix this with essential oils which are specifically good for the skin. Whey is excellent for the skin, outside as well as inside.

PERSPIRATION

Profuse sweating is one of the most important healing mechanisms known. In olden times people knew many more ways of producing sweat than we do today. Many sick people who have diabetes, arthritis, rheumatic diseases or cancer perspire only seldom and would benefit tremendously if they could perspire regularly. In the seventeenth century the well-known physician Sylvius said that 'one-third of all diseases could be healed by perspiration'.

Unfortunately there are fewer and fewer people who are able to perspire and many old means of inducing perspiration have been lost. Formerly doctors knew, for example, about a certain gold compound, which helped arthritis patients very much and was far less dangerous than the gold injections, which are used today. It was called *mercurius fixtus cum aurum*. Paracelsus knew many remedies that improved perspiration and were based on saltpetre (potassium nitrate), iron or sodium bicarbonate. Plant remedies like hawthorn, beech, lime and dandelion leaves and juniper berries were used to support perspiration and kidney functioning.

Locally applied humid and warm compresses, hot air treatment and the 'perspiration box;, a box with built-in light bulbs, were also used. This box was put over the patient as he or she lay flat in bed and patients who hardly ever perspired would start to sweat. Also sauna treatments and Turkish baths, as well as the warming baths of Maria Schlenz, were used. These methods were very successful in raising the body temperature. Fever therapy can still be of great help. In the case of cancer, for example, the temperature would be slowly increased to almost 42 degrees Celsius in order to destroy cancer cells. Nowadays this is achieved by hyperthermia treatment.

Most success has been achieved by combining perspiration therapies with excretory therapies in the following way. For two days before the treatment the patient eats only vegetable soup or wheat jelly. On the third day enemas and herbal remedies are given to clean out the intestines, after which the patient takes a warm bath until perspiration begins. It is good to add sea salt, herbs and plant extracts to the bath water, in order to improve the healing qualities. After the bath, the water should be dried off only a little and while the patient's skin is still damp, he or she should be wrapped in a big sheet or towel, put to bed and covered with woollen blankets. At the patient's feet and on both sides there should be hot water bottles. If the patient is not too weak he or she can continue perspiring for half an hour or longer. Afterwards the patient should be rubbed down with some diluted vinegar and then allowed to sleep for many hours. This kind of therapy has been known for thousands of years in many different variations.

Of course there are also many other ways in which to support perspiration, for instance with the help of exercises and other kinds of baths, packs or wraps. By means of perspiration many toxins are excreted directly through the skin and this kind of treatment is a wonderful experience, not only for the sick but also for healthy people.

When people perspire too much

When people perspire too much, especially when their hands perspire, it often has to do with a nervous disposition. Some people also perspire from physical weakness, if they have kidney problems or because they have eaten too much animal protein. Instead of using antiperspirants, which often contain substances that are dangerous for health, it is better to use Hamamelis soap from Bioforce, which contains witch hazel and thyme, and to take homeopathic drops like Salvia and Violaforce regularly. Also, homeopathic remedies like Silicea D12 are of great help.

The greatest danger when using antiperspirants lies in the fact that under the armpits or other places where the sweat comes out of the body, liquids can also get into the body. Lately breast cancer has been connected with different antiperspirants, as most breast cancer occurs in the upper and outside part of the breast.

CUPPING

Bloody cupping as well as dry cupping has been known since olden times. Dry cupping serves mainly to neutralise or offset inner congestion. If deep in the body too many toxins have been accumulating, it is possible by cupping to loosen these and bring them to the surface. Often there is an immediate alleviation of pain and inflammations at last get a chance to heal.

Generally this treatment is done with cupping glasses which now are also made from plastic. These cupping glasses are round cups in which either through heat or pressure a vacuum develops. The skin beneath this vacuum is sucked into the glass cup; unhealthy blood and toxins are brought to the surface and the inner organs are cleaned. Via the blood and lymph vessels the toxins are transported to the different excretory organs and can be excreted.

When the patient is strong and full-blooded, sometimes, depending on the disease, the physician will prescribe bloody cupping. In that case the skin is first scratched with a special instrument, so that during the cupping the cup will fill up with blood and through this blood many toxins will be excreted directly, instead of first passing through the excretory organs. The success of this method is based on the connections between the skin and the inner organs. This method is most successful when cupping in the area of the shoulders, the back or the neck.

When the physician notices some shallow dents in these areas, dry cupping is usually the best way, but if there are spongy or hard elevations on the skin, it is often better to use bloody cupping if the patient still has enough strength. In both methods, the skin, as well as the underlying tissues, the muscles, the nerves and the organs, which are connected with specific areas of the skin, are stimulated. Through cupping and many other methods one can stimulate the skin superficially and at the same time trigger off reactions deep in the body.

THE BAUNSCHEIDT METHOD

Outside of Germany, the Baunscheidt method is little known, although it was one of the most successful therapeutic methods of olden times. This method of bringing toxins from deep in the body to the surface is a real art. On the back, on the upper part of the arms and on other specific places there are areas which respond very well to the Baunscheidt method. There, the therapist, using a special instrument with very fine needles, makes tiny little holes and then rubs some special oil (Baunscheidt oil) into that part of the skin. Then the entire region is covered with cotton wool and not touched for about five days. Under the cotton wool small blisters or pustules appear which often rupture, so that they empty their contents into the cotton wool. This gives a light burning sensation.

During this treatment, toxins will not only be excreted, but also the very fine nerves under the skin will be stimulated. Therefore this method is often used in cases of diseases of the nerves, for example for very painful diseases like shingles. It is also possible to stimulate the function of weak organs and to influence many body processes in a positive way.

A Baunscheidt treatment for asthmatic complaints or bronchitis can bring much relief. This treatment has been very helpful in many different diseases and is one of the treatments that definitely should be taught at university.

CANTHARIDAL PLASTERS
It is no fairy tale that in olden times physicians could heal diseases which now seem to be incurable. There really were such cures and one of the reasons was that physicians did not treat their patients in such a circumspect way as today. They often used quite painful therapies like cauterisation (burning) and similar treatments. These treatments were often very successful, as many toxins were destroyed on the spot, so to speak, and the disease at last had a chance to heal. Patients in those days were less sensitive than we are now; today we are used to taking painkillers right away. Partly because of this many excellent therapies that were popular in the past are not used any more. However, many people are beginning to realise that the old ways were not so bad after all and one by one old treatments are being tried out again with much

success. One of the things which has now come back is the cantharidal plaster, which is made – ready for use – by a German pharmaceutical company.

Although this therapy resembles these excellent old therapies, it is not painful. The cantharidal plaster can be cut in such a way that it covers the place where one feels pain under the skin or deeper. There might be sciatic pains, muscle pains, stabbing pain and so on. Most of the time in places where one feels such pain there is an accumulation of toxins and these toxins have to be removed as soon as possible. A piece of cantharidal plaster, which sometimes is no bigger then a stamp, will be put on the skin and will then be covered completely with some dressing material and sealed with sticking plaster.

Under this plaster real miracles happen, and often after only a few hours light or even severe pain may disappear, for example in the knees or in the back. At the same time in this area a blister develops and this blister contains acids and lymphatic fluid, which were the main causes of the pain. It is best to leave the plaster in place for about 20 hours. Then the blister should be opened carefully with a fine needle, so that the liquid can run out. This little wound will heal in a few days. When the wound is bigger it will take about a week to heal. As this plaster helps when there is pain deeper in the body, it often seems a real miracle when such a pain disappears and it is inexplicable that only a few physicians know about the treatment. It is complete nonsense to treat such pain with creams or pills for a long time, when by using these plasters or other natural treatments instead the pain could disappear in hours or days.

CHAPTER FIVE

Healing via the Bloodstream

Bloodletting

Please note: bloodletting is a very exact art. Only physicians who are very experienced in the therapy should use it.

In the past, bloodletting was one of the most important treatments for many diseases. In primeval times healers opened different blood vessels with thorns, sharp little stones or bone splinters. This treatment was and still is used in Egyptian and Indian medicine and Hippocrates taught his pupils how, in this way, pneumonia, coronaries and many other diseases could be cured and prevented. Sydenham, Hufeland and Galen regarded bloodletting as an indispensable part of medicine. In the Middle Ages even the monks used bloodletting in order to prevent illness or as a treatment for illness. In medical literature there are many references about the often lifesaving effects of bloodletting.

The physicians of olden times observed nature and supported all the natural defensive measures of the body, such as spontaneous bleeding, in every possible way. Haemorrhoids were called 'the golden veins' and it was known that such bleedings should not be suppressed immediately. Haemorrhoids, especially those that are bleeding, relieve local blood pressure and when there is congestion in the legs and the pelvic organs they function as a valve, as they do also when there is an ulcus cruris (varicose ulcer), and many toxins are excreted in this way. When such a valve is closed too soon, it can have serious consequences. Nosebleeds, bleeding of the gums and of course menstruation all have the purpose of thoroughly cleaning the organism.

In summer when you see all those buses full of elderly tourists, you will notice that the majority of these tourists are women. Most of them will have lost their husbands not only as the result of too much stress, but mainly because men do not have the opportunity to clean their blood every month! Women are lucky, as during the best years of their life, every month a certain amount of old blood is excreted, and within only a few days new blood, free from toxins, is produced. With the old blood many toxic substances leave the body and the new blood is pure and healthy. When the monthly period stops, the blood often becomes thick and sometimes blockages occur. Consequently many women then suffer from different health problems. The best method to prevent or at least alleviate most of these problems is a regular bloodletting.

When people are still young and healthy, their blood has a nice red colour and is quite liquid. When people become old and sick their blood changes. During bloodletting this shows very clearly. Such blood is often thick, tough and very dark in colour and has the tendency to coagulate quickly. The condition of the blood has to do with its protein content and other factors, which always depend on the nutrition, the way of living and the general health of the person in question.

As far back as the sixteenth century Botallis spoke about the wonderful results of bloodletting. He said, 'The more impure water is pulled out of a well, the more clean water will flow back into this well.' This can be proved when an elderly person undergoes a course of bloodletting. With each treatment the blood of the patient becomes visibly cleaner. This is the best, most simple and completely harmless way to normalise high blood pressure! However, writing a presciption gives much less work and pays better!

Many diseases could be prevented and cured by regular bloodletting and this is logical, as the blood nourishes all body cells. Only pure and healthy blood can guarantee a healthy body. Thousands of documents from the past show the success of bloodletting, for example in cases of concussion of the brain, bleeding of the kidneys, fractures in the base of the skull and pulmonary embolism. It is very sad that modern medicine has apparently forgotten all about the wonderful healing possibilities of bloodletting. In the case of some very serious diseases, especially infectious diseases, for which modern physicians prescribe strong and harmful medication, bloodletting could often help much faster and better.

If bloodletting is so good, how can the attitude of modern physicians be explained? Why is such an excellent therapy, which has been known for thousands of years, not taught at university? This is in the first place due to the fact that in the eighteenth and nineteenth centuries doctors loved bleeding their patients so much that they sometimes overdid it. They did not yet know how much blood the human body contained and when too much blood was taken their patients died. As many of their patients were members of the nobility, who paid much money for bloodletting, this practice fell into disrepute. In the second place people nowadays believe that bloodletting is an old-fashioned and primitive treatment, which no longer belongs to our modern time and of course the pharmaceutical industry is very much against bloodletting, as this practice would interfere with much very lucrative business. This, however, is a great therapeutic loss, as bloodletting, especially for the diseases of our modern civilisation, is a wonderful means of treatment. Although formerly some physicians took too much blood from their patients, the best physicians never did this; they always knew exactly what they were doing and their achievements were very impressive.

In former times doctors not only took blood from the inside of the elbow joint, as they do now, but also from the ears, from under the tongue, from the knee joint and so on. Depending on the kind of disease they cut the skin superficially or deeper with a short or longer incision.

In the case of concussions or bone fractures an immediate bloodletting is the best way to prevent complications and more serious damage and in an emergency every physician should know how to do this. Even if the patient has no complaints after an accident, it would be advisable to let just a small amount of blood. Often after an accident a little blood remains in the brain which cannot be seen on the X-ray screen and if after some time this blood has not been absorbed, it could cause increasing pressure in the head. The consequences could be rather bad.

Babies sometimes fall on their heads when they are still very small and there are also parents who make a habit of slapingp their children on the head. In both cases there could be bruises or bleeding somewhere in or near the brain, which could cause migraines or other serious problems later in life. In folk medicine such haemorrhages are often dissolved using pure olive oil. In places where the head is very sensitive the oil is rubbed in and massaged very gently twice a day for some minutes, over the course of a few weeks or even months. Olive oil is the only kind of oil that can penetrate into the hardest stones. Only olive oil is able to dissolve blood clots, which are located under the skin and the cranial bones.

The fact that bloodletting is hardly used any more nowadays has had very serious consequences. The well-known physician Bernard Aschner said that this 'certainly has cost millions of human lives'. We can only hope that more physicians will become interested in using this therapy.

GENERAL USES FOR BLOODLETTING ARE:

1. For the thinning of the blood. This is the best way to treat high blood pressure.
2. To clear infections.
3. To detoxify and clean the blood.
4. To stimulate the excretion of toxins.
5. For relief from cramps or pain.
6. During the menopause (change of life) bloodletting helps in relieving hot flushes, depression, dizziness and headaches.
7. If somebody has skin that becomes easily bruised or bluish, this can often be healed by one or two bloodlettings.
8. Bloodletting helps greatly in the case of haemorrhoids.
9. Blood in the urine often disappears after one bloodletting.
10. Migraine, sleeplessness, sweating, ringing in the

ears, bleeding of the nose and the retina of the eye, shortness of breath, pleurisy and hepatitis can be alleviated by bloodletting and may sometimes even be cured in this way.

11. In the case of chronic diseases like rheumatic diseases, skin diseases, too little urine and so on, the blood should be cleaned by regular bloodlettings of small quantities of blood, about 120 to 200 ccm.

As harmful and irritating substances are eliminated through bloodletting and a general new adjustment takes place in the body, it is often far superior to most medication.

With this treatment you will not have to worry about losing too much blood or becoming anaemic; that is not possible. Nowadays because of ignorance and prejudice physicians often make a big mistake when they declare diseases, which could be much improved by bloodletting or other forgotten treatments, to be 'incurable'. A physician who has once known the healing effect of this therapy will continue using bloodletting whenever it is needed. Also, it is good to know that it has no side effects!

Spontaneously Produced Bleeding

Spontaneous bleeding is always a defence reaction of the organism. It acts as a valve, thereby preventing all kinds of congestion.

NOSEBLEEDS

A sudden bleeding from the nose can prevent cerebral bleeding or a stroke. In this case the surplus of blood is diverted and comes out through the nose. It is often wrong and could even be life-endangering to stop this bleeding immediately. Nosebleeds can develop because of local or general blockages, or may be the consequence of an accumulation of mucous after a cold, or because of adenoids, which also cause blockages.

If nosebleeds last too long one can always try to divert the blood away from the head by taking a warm foot-bath. A cold compress on the neck can also help, and this should be exchanged several times for a fresh one. Some people use a cotton-wool swab soaked in a little water and vinegar, which they put in one nostril and then close the bleeding nostril wing. But you should never forget that nosebleeds can often be just as healthy as bloodletting and that they can prevent serious health problems. Therefore it is best to let the blood run out for some time. Often a bleeding nose can give great relief and sometimes it cures tension and headaches within a short time. The Greek physician Athenaios, who prescribed bloodletting, would provoke nosebleeds as part of treatment.

RETINAL DETACHMENT
The dreaded detachment of the retina is mainly due to bleeding behind the eyes. This kind of problem is caused either by high blood pressure or by local blockage of the blood flow, as well as through overexertion. This can be prevented by regular blood donation, bloodletting and/or by biological treatments. If there is high interocular pressure and danger of retinal detachment, one should as soon as possible have a bloodletting. This prevents further development of the problem and can never do any harm.

Bleeding under the skin (bruises)

Little, or more extensive, bleeding under the skin, as well as bluish spots are usually caused by local blockages in the tissues, by weak connective tissues or by capillaries that have been damaged by toxins. Such problems could be prevented by a change of diet and a biological treatment. A lack of certain vitamins (A, B and F) can weaken the tissues and the walls of the capillaries so that they become porous. Bleeding of the gums is often caused by a lack of vitamin C and too much blood in the body. Such bleedings are called vicarious (substituted) bleedings.

Bleeding from the uterus

So-called benign uterus bleeding, which sometimes occurs after the menopause, is treated nowadays by radiation, hormones or even by a radical operation. Formerly such bleedings were treated by bloodletting, enemas and laxatives. They are often caused by local congestion (blockage) or, according to Bernard Aschner, by certain toxins. Elderly women who suffer from such bleeding often have a high blood pressure.

When younger women lose too little blood when menstruating, or when they do not menstruate at all for some time, this can be due to a spasmodic state whereby they do not excrete enough toxins. When these toxins accumulate somewhere in the body, they can be the cause of physical, as well as mental, problems.

After a radical operation, there is an artificial menopause. Regular bloodletting is extremely important for these women, because in that way many health problems can be prevented. If a woman does not menstruate anymore and there is no more monthly cleaning of the blood, she should try to perspire as much as possible. Constipation should be cured as soon as possible by a change of diet and by natural remedies.

HAEMORRHOIDS (BLEEDING PILES)
Haemorrhoids are also natural bloodlettings by which serious diseases can be prevented. They are never a local problem, but are usually caused by high blood pressure, overeating, refined foods, too little exercise or because of an abuse of laxatives. When these haemorrhoids are operated on, the cause of the problem is not removed. Such a treatment is only symptomatic.

Haemorrhoids can be caused by chronic constipation or by a habitual suppression of the stool; in that case blockages in the area of the rectum develop. Also a weakness of the connective tissues or a lack of fibre in the diet can provoke congestion of the portal vein, the liver and the gall bladder, so that haemorrhoids are pressed to the outside.

Haemorrhoids are a widespread ailment. A change of diet, more exercise, the treatment of constipation, cooling hip-baths, bloodletting and natural remedies that support the liver and the gall bladder can help. Different hydro-therapeutic treatments (water treatments) have a relaxing effect on the muscles of the anus. Often two to three times a week a cold hip-bath of eight to ten seconds will be prescribed. Thereafter the patient should get into a warm bed or go for a walk.

When treating haemorrhoids, the sanitation of the intestinal flora is a must; at the same time constipation should be cured. Strong laxatives should always be avoided. It is better to use Glauber's salt (*natrium sulphuricum*), bitter salts, cream of tartar or linseed.

Folk medicine still uses local treatments, with tannic acid from plants, for example from the bark of oaks or chestnuts. Now there are many biological ointments, suppositories and creams that contain tannic acid. Cherries, blackberries and blueberries contain pigments which strengthen the muscles of the anus and decrease the swelling. The juice from these berries mixed with apple juice, besides helping the problem also tastes very good and is a rather cheap and effective remedy.

Homeopathic remedies are for example Aesculus D6 or Hamamelis D3. Castor oil softens the haemorrhoids. Lumbar compresses with vinegar water three times a week are used in folk medicine, and alternate warm and cold compresses are also used. Finally I would like to mention the potato stoppers of Dr Jensen. These are cut from raw potatoes and the end should be rounded. Then they should be soaked in a little oil before inserting them in the anus. This should be done at night. With the next stool they come out again. They bring great relief.

Leeches

Although many people do not like to use or even look at them, leeches have helped a great many people in ancient times and also in our time. They are very effective and totally harmless. Leeches make a small hole in the skin and through this hole they absorb the diseased blood. But that is not all. In the saliva of these leeches there are very specific enzymes that dilute and detoxify the blood, so that the connective tissues are cleaned and healed.

In the case of venous stasis and inflammation, *ulcus cruris* (open legs), diseases of the eyes, ringing of the ears, dizziness and so on, one can witness real miracle cures when using leeches.

CHAPTER SIX

Hydrotherapy

All natural therapies aim at breaking up, dissolving, transporting and excreting toxins that threaten the health of the organism and hinder the normal bodily processes. Hippocrates was very interested in hydrotherapy. He knew the different effects of hot and cold water treatments and often prescribed baths, compresses and enemas. Paracelsus (*c*. 1493–1541) travelled from spa to spa and prescribed bath treatments. Vincent Priessnitz (1794–1851) cured thousands of patients with water cures. He used to combine perspiration and cold water treatments. Sebastian Kneipp (1821–1897) combined herbal treatments with an ingenious form of hydrotherapy. Dr Max Bircher-Benner (1867–1939) often prescribed Kuhne's baths and other treatments of hydrotherapy.

In the year 1886, after the book *The New Science of Healing* by Louis Kuhne had been published, his book was translated into 28 languages in 130 editions. This book, which is still on the market, deals with very specific bath treatments, with sunbathing and Turkish baths. He became world-famous; innumerable people read his books and were healed by his treatments. Other well known or even famous 'water doctors' were, amongst others, Rickli, Just, Fielke, Antonio Musa, Charms, Wright, Currie, Halm, Fleury, Winternitz, Maria Schlenz and Perez. Fleury was the director of a scientific school for hydrotherapy.

When a therapist uses massage or physiotherapy, many toxins in the body are broken up, dissolved and then go into the lymph channels or the circulating blood, after which they can be excreted from the body. While in massage the toxins will only be moved elsewhere within the body, in hydrotherapy or when a patient perspires toxins often leave the body in a direct way through the pores of the skin.

As an immediate reaction to the warm temperature of the water, the pores of the skin will open. When using cold water, at first the opposite effect occurs; the pores close and the blood vessels near the surface of the skin contract. Thus the blood flows into blood vessels which are located deeper in the body. In this way the blood circulation around the vital organs improves and toxins which have been accumulating, sometimes for years, get into the general blood circulation. In the meantime the initial contraction of the outer skin diminishes and the blood vessels which are located right under the skin open and take up toxins which originally were deep in the body. These toxins can now be excreted via the pores of the skin. As a consequence the blood vessels under the skin will be well supplied with blood and this explains the warm feeling after a cold shower.

In former times most 'water doctors' used cold water treatments almost exclusively. Nowadays people are very spoiled. They often feel cold and only seldom experience the desirable warming effect of a cold-water treatment. It can happen that a patient feels even colder after such a treatment. These so-called 'spastic patients' need warm instead of cold treatments and the spa doctor will try to normalise the reaction of these patients by 'hardening' them.

It would be impossible to discuss all possible water treatments in this chapter. There are many books on the subject which describe most of the treatments used today in great detail. However, some of the most interesting and successful treatments are mentioned only seldom. Here I will try to make up for this.

Priessnitz

Let us go back to Priessnitz. He treated chronic, as well as some acute, diseases, with hydrotherapy combined with other natural treatments. He said that the patient should always drink enough water and he prescribed rest, warmth and simple food. Before starting the treatment he ordered enemas in order to empty and clean the colon.

Unlike his predecessors he combined perspiration with water cures. The more people perspired before a bath, the better they felt afterwards. Perspiring stimulated the heart, but the bath afterwards had a calming effect. If patients were very old or weak Priessnitz did not apply these tiring treatments. He refused to treat patients suffering from tuberculosis, liver diseases cancer, or very weak patients.

Fresh air, exercise and massage were very important in his clinic and a treatment he often used was the 'Neptune belt'. This was a humid abdominal compress, which was tightly covered with a dry cloth and worn under the clothes, sometimes all day long.

Priessnitz prescribed cleaning and strengthening the intestinal tract, and cold baths and compresses were alternated with perspiration and rubbing the body. During this treatment the symptoms of the disease worsened first of all. The aim was to develop skin rashes (cutaneous eruptions) and sometimes the patient suffered from a high temperature. When this happened, even if there was much pain, once the healing crisis was achieved the toxins could leave the body and the patient could be cured. In that case the treatment was continued and after some time the skin rash disappeared along with the disease. From all over the world people came to be treated by Priessnitz. No wonder, because his results were excellent.

In the time of Priessnitz there were about 80 such water clinics in Germany. Their directors were mainly physicians who had trained with Priessnitz. In 1846, 5,000 patients were treated in his clinic.

All Day Long in the Bathtub

When we have to take a bath for half an hour, often this demands much of our time and patience. However, in some parts of the world people used to bathe for hours and sometimes for days. In Japan, Mexico and even in Europe, people who went to a spa often stayed for a long time in the water, as this was part of the treatment.

In Mexico, healing herbs, sea salt or oil and sometimes sweet-smelling essences were often added to the water; such baths were very soothing and relaxing. The old Mexican schools produced excellent physicians. They mainly used two different kinds of treatment that complemented each other, hydrotherapy and aromatherapy, which is still very popular. In Japan hot baths have always been used. Erwin Bälz, the author of the book *The Life of a German doctor in the Awakening Japan*, lived in Tokyo for many years. He wrote: 'The temperature of the bath is never below 40 degrees Celsius because experience has proved that people easily catch a cold if the temperature is lower. Before entering such a hot bath, people should always douse their head with hot water in order to prevent complications.' This was also customary in some European spas, as great variation in temperature in different parts of the body could result in fainting or worse problems.

Today, in Japan people are still accustomed to taking baths very often; they do this at home or they use public baths. They do this not only in order to be clean, but also for health reasons. In Japan it is still quite normal to take a bath that lasts some hours or sometimes even a few days. In Europe too, until the First World War, bathing was a form of therapy, which many well-known physicians like Leyden, Leube and Ziemissen prescribed. August Heissler describes Duke William of Saxony's visit to the spa of Wildbad in 1436. The duke stayed in the bath for eight or nine hours every day.

In the middle of the sixteenth century many people went to the spa of Karlsbad in Bohemia, where they also took baths of very long duration. They started this therapy with one hour in the morning and one in the afternoon. After this they stayed in the water every day for one hour more until they spent eight to ten hours a day in the bath. These cures were still short compared to the thermal baths of Kawanaka in Japan, which Dr Bälz described. Here, some people stayed day and night in the water, sometimes even for weeks.

I quote August Heissler:

> On the 13th of April 1737 Georg Friedrich
> Händel, the well-known composer, had a stroke
> while living in London. This stroke resulted in his
> right side becoming paralysed and his ability to
> speak curtailed. As there was no improvement
> after five months, his doctors sent him for a bath
> treatment to Aachen in Germany. The physicians
> in Aachen allowed him to stay in a warm bath for
> three hours a day, but despite strict warnings that
> this could be fatal, he stayed in the water for nine
> hours a day. After only a week he could already
> drag himself to the bath, after the second week he
> was able to move his paralysed arm and on the
> last day of his treatment he climbed the steps to
> the church in Aachen to play the organ.

We are very lucky that at that time this kind of treatment
was available and that Händel had more courage than all
his physicians. Otherwise, we would be short of three of
Händel's best operas!

Horst Muller wrote in his book *Water Treatments for
Healthy People and for Patients* about a 'neutral bath'.
This was a full bath to which new hot water was
constantly added. The duration of this bath was between
one and six hours and caused a profound relaxation of all
the body muscles. Unfortunately, in our time only a few
people know the wonderful healing effect of such a bath.

If the water stays at the same temperature, after about
three hours it will already begin to penetrate deep into
the body, so that many toxins are dissolved and
eliminated. Formerly many diseases and even some kinds
of paralysis were treated and healed in this way.

The Bath Cure of Maria Schlenz

Mrs Maria Schlenz was a well-known therapist, who first treated herself and later her relatives and patients with a bath therapy which lasted for several hours. She had often observed that the temperature of the body adjusted by and by to the temperature of the water and she raised the water temperature slowly to 38 degrees Celsius, and in the case of cancer patients to over 40 degrees. In order to prevent the head getting too cool, her patients always had to wear a woollen cap when taking a bath. She used a little wooden board to support the head of the patients and the water came up to their nose. This kind of therapy was very successful in the treatment of diseases of the head and the ears.

Later, Maria Schlenz began to use water temperatures of 36 to 37 degrees to start with, raising the temperature to 39 degrees within 20 minutes. After the temperature had gone down again to 38 degrees, it was kept this way until the end of the bath. Such bath cures can obtain very good results when used to treat rheumatic and circulatory diseases. The temperature and the duration of the cures depend on the strength of the patient's immune system, the kind of disease and other factors.

Once in a while during a course of these bath cures a patient may undergo 'healing reactions', which are very positive as they indicate that harmful substances are being detoxified and eliminated. Healing reactions include, for example, nausea, an urge to pass water, weeping eyes, headaches, depression and so on. Such reactions last only for a short time and should never be suppressed. Sometimes just taking a deep breath or brushing the skin while in the bath may help, as well as drinking some mint tea, or tea made with speedwell, horsetail, chamomile or St John's Wort. Even a cup of coffee can be beneficial, as in this case the beverage is used as a remedy. It is completely normal that a patient may feel a little weak or dizzy when leaving the bath. During the cure there can also be increased perspiration. It should always be remembered that it is not the cure itself which weakens the patient; the weakness and other symptoms are mainly due to the excretion of toxins.

Interrupting or even ending the treatment before a cure is finished can be very dangerous, as in that case all the toxins which have been broken down and are now in the bloodstream are suddenly prevented from being eliminated. In such cases, there will be strong and often dangerous reactions. In our time, physicians who do not understand anything about the healing reactions discussed above could misinterpret these and by ending the cure right away they might even endanger the life of the patient.

If the patient suffers from constipation, it is necessary to clean out the intestines before the bath cure. This cure also can be supported, as the Mexican physicians used to do, by massaging the body with essential oils. It is not advisable to fast during the cure; some light and healthy food will be best.

Whenever possible, sea water should be used. Many mineral springs contain salts that are often too highly concentrated, and are either too acid or too alkaline. Sea water has more or less the same composition as our blood; therefore we can assimilate minerals from the sea easily into our body. If there is no sea water available sea salt or herbal extracts can be added to the water. When patients are too weak to tolerate a long and tiring bath cure, they can take a bath of shorter duration, with the temperature slowly increased, every evening for as long as they need it. After the bath, they should be wrapped up in a warm towel and sleep in a warm bed all night. In this way, even patients who are very weak can be helped.

Not only Maria Schlenz but also many other well known physicians have used this kind of treatment for their patients. According to Dr Eisenberg, 'water always has the effect of an absorbent tampon which drains toxins out of the body'. A famous doctor who treated many patients in this way was Dr Nahmacher, who because of these cures often prevented amputations, *ulcus cruris*, and even paralysis.

Sebastian Kneipp

Sebastian Kneipp was one of the great pioneers of health reform at the end of the nineteenth century. With his great knowledge and understanding of the laws of nature and of herbal remedies, he was able to help thousands of ill and suffering people. Today his healing methods are world-famous. He was convinced that modern people get too little light and sunlight and have too little contact with water. In his opinion, illness develops when the organism is weak and has too little resistance. He said that people need plenty of exercise and a constant supply of natural stimuli in order to harden the body and in former times this was a matter of course. Modern people are too spoilt and pampered and because of this their defence mechanisms have weakened. The more drastic healing measures of olden times can no longer be applied, as in general patients today do not have enough courage and strength to tolerate these.

According to Kneipp, many diseases are caused by genetic disorders of the glands, the nerves or the blood vessels. However, even if a person has the disposition for a certain disease, he or she will only develop this disease if the defensive forces are low.

Already Kneipp was convinced that the fear of germs was much exaggerated. Similar to plants, germs need the right environment and nutrients in order to grow. Harmful germs will only multiply if the blood and body tissues of the host (the person in question) are unhealthy. Therefore Kneipp believed it was only possible to cure a patient after their blood was cleaned and their eating habits were changed. Every Kneipp treatment was based on a correct diet and on the simultaneous strengthening of weak organs and other body parts. As all healing procedures depend on the condition of the excretory organs, he encouraged perspiration. If the patient could not perspire properly he applied methods to encourage profuse perspiration. Some of his baths and wet packs can be life-saving.

Through hydrotherapy more toxins can be excreted in the urine. Water inside and outside the body can stimulate a better evacuation of the bowels. In this way, headaches, pressure on the brain and nervous tension can disappear surprisingly quickly. During these hydrotherapeutic treatments, there can be temporary signs of an acute illness with inflammation, skin rashes and/or fever. Fever is one of the best remedies; only if it is very high and lasts for more than three days should it be lowered by natural methods.

The duration and type of treatment always depends on the strength of the natural defence mechanism of each patient; some patients need stimulating while others need soothing measures. Each kind of treatment has a different effect on the excretion of toxins and blood circulation. Kneipp was the first therapist to create adaptable treatments which gradually strengthened the immune system. The immune system may be stimulated by cold, but in this case the physician should supervise the patient very carefully. The great variety of the Kneipp treatments makes it possible to help patients of any age group. His therapies strengthen the defensive forces of the body and can be applied to treat the majority of diseases without restrictions.

It was Sebastian Kneipp who masterminded a well-ordered system out of the almost chaotic variety of hydrotherapeutic treatments of his time. Although his system of treatment was designed with scientific accuracy, it was never dogmatic.

It would be impossible to describe all the different Kneipp treatments and recipes in this book. However, anybody interested in his healing ways can buy books about the Kneipp therapy, which are published worldwide.

The Successful and Unique Healing Ways of Louis Kuhne

Louis Kuhne was born in Leipzig in 1840. From his parents he had inherited a weak constitution and he was often ill. Innumerable physicians treated him as a child and when he was a young man, but nobody managed to cure him; so he decided to cure himself. He felt sure that alien substances were the cause of all diseases. These substances accumulated in the body and the most important thing was to somehow rid the body of them.

In the second half of the nineteenth century people became more and more interested in the nervous system. It was known that numerous nerve-ends and nerves in the lower body were in some way connected with vital organs and other parts of the body. Louis Kuhne's idea was that most diseases were caused by fermentation of foreign substances, especially in the lower regions of the body, and that if he could stop this fermentative process he could cure illness.

As people already knew in that time that fermentation could be stopped by cold, Louis Kuhne cured himself with cold water. He invented a cold water treatment, whereby the patient washes the lower parts of his or her body for some time with cold water in order to promote blood circulation and the excretion of toxins. The treatment varies for men and women.

How Kuhne's treatment is done by women
One fills a bidet, or a bucket over which a wooden board has been placed, with cold water. In preparation a body brush should be covered with a cloth, or flannel. The patient then sits on the board or bidet and, continuously dipping the brush into the cold water, washes the lower part of the body, especially the genitals, from top to bottom. To begin with this should be done for 5–10 minutes 2 or 3 times a day and should then be increased to 20–30 minutes daily. During this treatment the rest of the body should always be kept warm and the patient should wear woollen socks and slippers.

After the treatment the patient should get into a warm bed or go for a walk. In summer or when living in a warm climate, some ice cubes should be put into the water to make sure it is cold enough.

How Kuhne's treatment is done by men
The treatment is similar for men. They should carefully wash the foreskin under the water with a cloth. During

this treatment a rash may occur on the outer genitalia. This is normal and is usually a sign that in this region many toxins have accumulated. This therapy can also be done in a more modern way by using a hand-shower, which is moved slowly over the genitalia.

Louis Kuhne himself was completely healed by his own therapy and he treated thousands of patients who suffered from many different diseases in the same way. He was internationally known and was so successful that his book, *The New Science of Healing* (*Die Neue Heilwissenschaft*), has at the time of writing reached 130,000 editions and has been translated into 28 languages. In this book he also describes several other natural healing methods.

After him other famous physicians and healers took over his curative methods and not long ago even Dr Max Bircher-Benner prescribed this therapy for his patients in his clinic in Zurich, Switzerland.

CHAPTER SEVEN

Reflexology

Neural Therapy

Ferdinand and Walter Huneke were two brothers who in the year 1925 discovered a new kind of treatment, which since then has cured many thousands of people suffering from severe pain, paralytic symptoms and other health problems. They had a sister, who for many years had suffered from very severe migraine headaches. Both brothers were physicians; they had tried everything in order to help their sister, but nothing changed her condition. One day Ferdinand gave her by mistake an intravenous injection which contained an anaesthetic called 'procaine'; this anaesthetic should never have been injected into a vein. At that moment his sister's headache disappeared and never came back. After this success both brothers tested the medicament, first being their own guinea pigs before using it on their patients. They also discovered that the addition of a little caffeine made the injections of procaine even more efficient. In the year 1928 they published their first results in the magazine *Medical World* under the title 'Unknown Remote Action of Local Anaesthetics'. They spent the rest of their lives researching and studying the different healing effects of procaine.

Even when procaine was not injected directly into the vein but next to it, the treatment was successful. This proved that the healing was not only achieved via the bloodstream, but also via the nerves. Later Ferdinand and Walter discovered that all illness and healing is controlled by the nervous system.

Many people know that the success of acupuncture and reflexology is based on certain energy streams in the organism. Everything alive has energy continuously flowing throughout the organism. If at some point in the body this energy flow is interrupted, it can sometimes have serious consequences, which can occur in a completely different part of the body.

To be able to understand this, one has to imagine an electrical circuit to which many light bulbs are connected. If one day one of these light bulbs does not burn any more the fault may be in the light bulb itself, or somewhere else quite a distance away in the wires or in the wall socket. The same applies to the human body. Yet many physicians do not understand that the original cause of pain, inflammation or even some paralytic problems often lies elsewhere in the body.

A physician who has had experience with neural therapy has to know about all the possible places in the body of his patient where the energy flow could have been interrupted, and will ask the patient all kinds of questions in order to find this out. The slightest incident could cause a possible disorder. In particular, any scar from a tonsillectomy or an appendix operation, or even a small cut in a finger, can block the energy stream. Often little scars on the head or in the ears (after an ear infection) in early childhood can be responsible for serious health problems later on. Sometimes scars may be dormant for years and when later they become hard and lose their elasticity, they obstruct the energy flow. This explains why some kinds of paralysis for example develop only gradually.

Practitioners of neural therapy treat many different diseases by specific injections in all the places that might be responsible for an obstruction in the energy flow. Procaine or a similar anaesthetic will be injected into all the scars with a very fine needle, especially if these scars still hurt a little. It can happen that after such an injection many health problems disappear all of a sudden and at the same time. But most often several treatments and more injections will be needed.

There is also 'segmental therapy', whereby many small injections are given in a certain section of the skin which corresponds with the place where the symptoms are. If the problem disappears right away at the time of the first injection, this is called the 'sekunden phänomen' (a phenomenon which happens within seconds). This is a real miracle, which only happens once in a while.

Neural therapy is a wonderful therapy which the physician can often use to prevent an operation or cure a disease that did not respond to any other treatment. It is astonishing that so few physicians know about this wonderful way of healing, for through it many patients would be spared much suffering and pain.

Unknown Reflex Therapies

Thousands of years ago, Chinese acupuncture was based on the fact that inner organs and other body parts could be influenced in a stimulating or soothing way through innumerable points on the skin. These points can be found in the outer skin and also in the mucous membranes. We all know or have heard about the reflexology of the feet, whereby pain, cramps and several diseases can be treated. Some of us also may have heard about ear acupuncture.

However there are many more ways in which reflexology can be used successfully. In the past, for example in the time of Hippocrates, physicians already knew a great deal about some of the amazing healing effects of the therapy. Their treatments were often painful and patients in our time would hardly be able to tolerate them. Formerly, some physicians treated patients by using a very thin red-hot iron wire, even in cases of paralysis. With this wire they touched specific points deep in the nose for just a few seconds, so that a tiny part of the mucous membrane was cauterised. The results were remarkable and even some serious health problems were cured.

As nowadays we are far too sensitive and do not have such a high tolerance of pain, some physicians found similar methods of treatment which are more acceptable to the modern patient. Today's 'nasal therapy' is much gentler than it was in the past. It is done with a thin metal stick wrapped in cotton wool. This is dipped into a mixture of specific essential oils and specific points inside the nose are touched for a very short time. Someone who suffers from a blocked nose or who often has headaches can treat himself in this way by using a little cotton bud and a mild mixture of essential oils. This often gives great relief.

The nose is a very sensitive and interesting part of the body. On the mucous membrane in all nasal passages, many reflex points can be found and every one of these points corresponds to some inner organ or body region. Often this treatment causes sneezing, which is a very positive reaction.

SNEEZING

Sneezing was used as a therapy for thousands of years. Unfortunately, the habit of taking snuff has gone out of fashion. Sneezing cleans the head and makes us think more clearly. It is a natural cleaning process, and although some people think it is bad manners to sneeze in company, it is very good for your health to sneeze once in a while. However, remember to hold a handkerchief before your nose, because bacteria can spread as far as six metres around you when you sneeze. So, please enjoy it, but remember it can be harmful for other people who are in close proximity.

In olden times many plants were known that could provoke sneezing, for example sneezewort (also known as sneezeweed) or the root of helliboris. Many indigenous people collected plants and herbs for that purpose, and there are many African tribes who still follow the custom today. Sneezing is still considered to be very healthy in Japan and China. Sneezing improves blood circulation in the head and often helps against muscle cramps and tension.

On the head, on the back and near the spinal column there are innumerable reflex points. Another reflex therapy that most physicians have never heard about is the 'mouth acupuncture' of Dr Gleditsch. He found that when the acupuncture points in the mouth are touched, they react more or less in the same way as those in the nose.

The Chinese also use acupuncture points on the head and in Germany there is a rather new therapy, whereby the anaesthetic injections of neural therapy are combined with homeopathic active substances. One or two millilitres at the most are injected into the most superficial layer of the skin at certain acupuncture points. These specific points correspond with diseased organs or parts of the body. The results are sometimes amazing and the treatment is not painful.

Recently acupuncture and neural therapy were officially recognised by traditional medicine. Let us hope that physicians will try to learn more about these wonderful healing ways.

CHAPTER EIGHT

Simple Health Problems

Inflammation and Fever are Defence Reactions

An inflammation, like fever, is one of the best defence reactions of the body. An inflammation begins when other defence mechanisms of the body are unable to excrete all the toxins and germs by way of the skin, the intestines, the kidneys, the lungs and the bloodstream.

When the first natural stage of excretion cannot take place in the usual ways, it will be followed by stronger reactions, such as fever or inflammation A localised inflammation somewhere in the body can be seen as a local fever. If somebody has a temperature, or fever, this can be seen as a general inflammation of the organism. Such an inflammation induces swelling, reddening, heat, pain, weakness and tiredness. During an inflammation many different kinds of defensive cells are put into action and in the centre of the inflammation unimaginably high temperatures can develop, so that toxins and germs will be 'burned'.

Inflammation and fever have the task of restoring the balance of the organism. When an infection cannot be cured by way of a local inflammation, a fever will develop. Then inflammation and fever together have to achieve what it is impossible for the inflammation to do by itself. Without the help of inflammation and fever many toxins and harmful micro-organisms would spread all over the body and trigger off serious and sometimes life-threatening conditions.

Inflammation and fever will usually disappear by themselves if one does not interfere with these natural defence measures. If necessary, the naturopath doctor will support these defensive reactions in every possible way. As long as there is a temperature the patient should not eat, as during this time any food intake would obstruct the healing process. The organism would not be able to assimilate the nutrients and the digestion of the food would squander much valuable energy, which is needed urgently for healing. The patient should only drink water, herbal tea or diluted fruit or vegetable juices, which he should drink slowly in sips.

It is always important that the excretion of toxins through the lungs should take its normal course, therefore the patient should be well covered up and the window should be open day and night. Plenty of oxygen is an important healing factor. Also, the regular cleaning of the intestines should not be omitted and the patient should be given enemas and drink special herbal teas for this purpose. If he or she is not too weak, intestinal baths can be recommended. The cleaning of the intestinal tract not only serves to remove food residues, but also helps to evacuate all toxins which have accumulated.

The excretion of toxins by way of the skin should always be supported. The patient should perspire each day for some time and he or she can stimulate perspiration by drinking special herbal teas, by warm baths and by other hydrotherapeutic measures mentioned in chapter four. Afterwards the entire body of the patient should be washed with lukewarm water and the patient should rest.

The most important task of the physician is to support and encourage the defence mechanisms of the organism. If there is too little fever, the physician, with the help of homeopathic or natural remedies, will be able to raise the temperature of the body so that many toxins can be destroyed. A good physician will carry out these measures while taking the special needs of the patient and the condition of his or her defence mechanisms into account. When based on experience, real healing will always be an art.

Chronic inflammations are often the consequence of the disastrous suppression of symptoms, which makes the excretion of toxins impossible. When inflammations are suppressed, they will spread their poisons and waste products through the blood and body tissues, sometimes over many years. Slight chronic inflammations, when ignored, are often a focus of disease. Day and night the bloodstream transports toxins to the weaker organs or body regions, where they will be deposited and do harm. If such toxins are accumulating in the joints there will be secondary inflammations after some time. The longer such an inflammation exists, the more difficult it will be to heal.

Intestinal Problems

When people are suffering from the diseases of modern society, they also suffer from some health problems connected with their digestive organs. Diseased intestines are at the root of many different diseases, although most of the time we do not realise this. In order to function well, all our body cells need nutrients which come from our food and only when the intestines are healthy can the necessary nutrients be assimilated. However, when there is something wrong with the intestines most nutrients cannot or can only partly be assimilated. In that case, many body cells starve and will eventually die.

If you sometimes feel a pressure in the stomach or suffer from constipation or diarrhoea, this is a sign that something is not well with your intestines. Often your tongue will be white and coated; it can also look yellowish or brown and in the morning especially you may have a bad taste in the mouth. The stool will smell bad, although the stool of a healthy person has almost no smell at all.

Normally the intestines are covered with a mucous membrane which is so sensitive that it has to be renewed every day. However, when an unhealthy diet is eaten, a normal mucous membrane cannot be rebuilt. In that case the mucous membrane will become quite porous and when the tiny filters in the intestinal wall are damaged by sharp and irritating substances, more and more toxins get into the blood and the surrounding tissues. Because of this, the liver will be much overtaxed in its detoxification work.

If the person in question suffers from chronic constipation, in addition to all the other problems, his or her intestines will be like a sewer and the organism will be poisoned from the inside. The danger of such self-poisoning via the intestines increases when there are fewer and fewer stools. There are people who can only go to the toilet every second, third or even fourth day. Sometimes it can even happen that the physician sees patients in his practice who 'cannot go' for ten days or even longer!

Constipation, diarrhoea and other intestinal problems and diseases are mainly caused by wrong nutrition. As long as the intestines are diseased no physician can really cure other diseases from which the patient is suffering. Therefore, in the case of any disease it is extremely important to first cure the intestinal problems and to sanitise the intestinal flora.

A SHORT SUMMARY OF HOW TO HEAL THE INTESTINES
The patient should eat only natural, healthy food, so that no further toxins can enter the body. In this respect a short fast can be recommended.

In order to heal the intestines, one of the best diets is a cereal jelly cure, whereby the jelly is made from wheat, barley or rye (no oats, because these may irritate the intestines). The cereals should be cooked for some hours and then passed through a sieve. The patient should eat this jelly three times a day and nothing else for as long as desired, until the intestinal problems have disappeared. He or she should eat very slowly, so that there is plenty of saliva to moisten the food. Between meals water or herbal teas, such as fennel or sage, with a little honey may be drunk.

To the cereal jelly a little honey may be added or, if one prefers a salty taste, some soy sauce or sea salt. In this way the diet does not become too boring. During this time the patient should take an enema every night and should also once in a while introduce a little natural oil (such as virgin olive oil) into the anus with a small rectal syringe. This kills bacteria and also prevents the drying out of the bowels. At the beginning of the treatment, the washing out of the intestines (intestinal lavage) in a medical practice will be a great help.

If possible the patient should rest each day after the

midday meal for at least half an hour and during this time he or she should use a humid wrap on the abdomen. This helps digestion and is very agreeable. In order to sanitise the bacterial flora in the intestines it is recommended to take Symbioflor (a Biosym product), which rebuilds a healthy intestinal flora, Colibiogen from Color something similar.

When the stool does not smell bad any more, the other complaints have also gone and the results of the medical check-up are satisfactory, the patient can carefully, step by step, start eating a simple diet to build up the strength.

For about three weeks one should eat a cereal or Bircher muesli in the morning, without any milk or milk products other than a little cream. One should always add a freshly grated apple, some lemon juice and soaked dried fruits. At midday one should eat a mixed salad (no vinegar!) to start with. Then one can eat a cereal dish – rice, millet or couscous – with steamed vegetables or potatoes in their skin with a little butter and sea salt. At night the meal should consist of a cereal soup, or some other cereal dish. For a change one can have some wholewheat bread, flatbread or Swedish Knäckebrot with butter and a little Vitam-R (a salty paste) or some honey.

After such a diet, one can start slowly to eat all kinds of healthy wholefoods. When one has sensitive intestines it would be advisable to eat in this way as often as possible. Do not forget to eat slowly and to chew well, so that there is enough saliva to dissolve the food. If the complaints return it is advisable to begin the cereal jelly cure again immediately and to persevere with it for some time. Such recurrent complaints often indicate that the person in question has changed his or her diet from one stage to another too soon. In order to really cure a serious intestinal disease one needs much time and patience. However, the method described here is the only way to get rid of many, often very serious, complaints.

By using strong medication or other methods the physician or therapist only fiddles around with the symptoms and the patient usually gets worse and stays ill until the end of his or her life.

The Common Cold, a Sore Throat and Similar Problems

The common cold, a sore throat, coughing and sneezing are part of the natural defensive reactions of our organism. Pressure in the head, headaches, sleeplessness or hoarseness are also often defensive reactions against toxins or too much stress.

These defensive reactions start when too many toxins from the environment or the food put a strain on the organism. This also happens when the person in question has a lack of minerals, has been exposed to cold or windy weather, has wet or cold feet or is suffering from mental or emotional strain. Under these circumstances almost anybody can catch the flu from someone else, because the flu virus feels very much at home in a weakened organism. When someone suffers frequently from colds or sore throats it is a sign that the defence mechanisms of the body are very low and have been overtaxed too often. If this happens to you, it is high time to have a good look at your lifestyle and daily habits in order to prevent becoming more ill. Most often the fault lies with the nutritional or living habits of the person in question and most people know themselves what they are doing wrong.

Either one changes the bad habits or one takes the risk of becoming seriously ill. However, some health problems can also be partly due to overwork, or mental or emotional strain. Unfortunately it is not possible to prevent everything, but people can avoid many diseases and usually it is their own fault when their defence mechanisms become overburdened, as is the case when they eat too many refined carbohydrates and milk products or consume too many soft drinks. No wonder that so many children forever seem to have a runny nose and often get ill. Although the stress at school and a lack of sleep often play a role, more often unhealthy nutrition and soft drinks are the main cause of these perpetual colds.

The habit of giving children something to drink before and during meals cannot be recommended. It is very bad indeed when children are given soft drinks or artificial fruit juices. These contain so many calories that children lose their appetites completely or become addicted to carbohydrates. Usually these children are either too thin or too fat and none of them is really healthy.

Apart from this, too many liquids will dilute the digestive juices and the food will not be properly absorbed. Here the parents can set a good example and they will also feel better when they get into the habit of not drinking while eating. The food will be chewed and digested much more effectively. After some time the whole family will feel better and healthier.

Food allergies, for example allergic reactions to milk and milk products, are to blame more and more for flu and similar illnesses, which are diseases of the lymphatic system. When the lymphatic defences are weakened one can easily catch a cold, or get a sore throat or the flu. Milk is the lymphatic fluid of the cow and therefore it seems logical that in the case of a disease of the lymphatic system, milk and milk products are not right for patients who often catch a cold or flu, or suffer from sore throats or earaches.

Lack of sleep and often going to bed late always has negative consequences. The same thing happens when people continuously work long hours without relaxing once in a while. Also personal problems, too much stress at work, lack of fresh air and exercise and many of the other things we have to cope with in our modern life can diminish the defensive forces of the body.

It is amazing and often incomprehensible that otherwise quite intelligent people and even physicians seem to be unable to think in a logical and independent way about these problems. A dogmatic and detailed way of thinking dominates and handicaps not only the thought patterns of today's medicine and science, but also those of the intelligent public. They cannot see the wood for the trees. Etiology, which means 'the cause behind the causes', should be easy to understand, but it is now covered up by detail and the opinions of many different people. If one stops paying attention to the opinion of others, suddenly it can happen that things are not complicated any more and that the natural connections become clear and understandable. One can see why etiology was so terribly important to physicians like Bircher-Benner. Only when one can link the cause and the therapy can one remove the actual root of the disease. There are innumerable illnesses, but there are only a few causes.

If you are often tired or often catch a cold, if you suffer from headaches, migraines, nervousness or other 'normal' health problems, you should start using your little grey cells, like the famous Hercule Poirot in the books by Agatha Christie. Most of the time you can discover the actual cause of these problems yourself, and then you can do something about them.

Obesity

Just like intestinal problems and the common cold, in general gaining too much weight belongs to the category of simple health problems, which, however, can have very serious consequences when neglected. Therefore it is very important to prevent real obesity, which is a metabolic disease. It is one of the most common diseases of Western society and in the last three or four decades has become an increasing danger for the health of the population.

The first people on earth were mainly vegetarian. Their nutrition consisted of natural carbohydrates, little fat and little protein. The fruit sugar (fructose) from the food was immediately assimilated and used for energy. Once in a while there was also a little glucose (grape sugar); with the help of insulin part of this glucose was deposited as body fat. In this way it was possible for these people to survive in times of hunger. Because all food was natural, metabolism usually proceeded normally. In olden times people had a lot of stamina and in general they were far stronger than we are. Such qualities are now mainly only found in some primitive peoples.

During the 'Neolithic Revolution' in about 5000 BC, nutritional habits were changing. By selecting different kinds of grasses, it became possible to cultivate some useful cereals. The cereal grains could be kept for a very long time and there was less need to go looking for food. People became used to a little more comfort and enjoyed cereals, which had a very seductive taste. Cereals were now eaten throughout the year in ever-greater quantities and this was too much work for the pancreas. Therefore even then there were already reports of obesity and diabetes amongst the rich upper classes in Mesopotamia and Greece, because these rich people did not do any hard work. Fortunately most people were used to doing a great deal of physical work, so that a great part of the different kinds of sugar from the cereals was used as energy.

In our time there are more and more people who are obese. In the industrial countries this has become almost endemic. Not only adults but also children are gaining far too much weight. There are several reasons for this; we eat too much, there is too much fat in our diets and daily we are inundated with refined carbohydrates which formerly did not exist. Most of these foods are stored in the body as fat. Besides this, we take too little exercise and mainly the older generation is happy if they can sit peacefully in front of their televisions.

Most overweight people are not really happy with their weight. However, it is very difficult to get rid of superfluous body fat and every overweight person knows about the 'Yo-Yo Effect'. This means that after every diet there is another weight gain and within a short time the weight of the person in question is the same again or even more than before. This is because the body, just like in times of famine, simply lowers its needs when there is less to eat, so that fewer calories are needed for every activity. Practically this means, for example, that formerly when the person in question swam for about 30 minutes he used up 150 calories, but now for the same performance he only needs about 120 calories. The organism goes on a low flame and when this person starts eating normally again the remaining calories are changed into body fat.

In *10 Golden Rules for Good Health* I wrote about the fact that Americans are very afraid to eat the slightest bit of fat. This gives us the impression that fat makes fat. Although this is partly true, it is hardly ever realised that some carbohydrates can be at least as dangerous as fat.

The tendency towards obesity often starts during childhood. When babies and small children are overfed this can have an effect on their eating habits throughout their lives. By eating sensibly themselves, parents can influence the future of their children in a positive way. A Japanese proverb says: 'Who loves his children beats them often, who hates his children gives them much to eat'. Fat cells which develop in childhood can always fill up again later in life. This occurs when the person in question eats the wrong kind of food, or too great a quantity.

Natural food is never fattening! In order to lose weight the best thing is to eat very simple, natural, wholesome food and once in a while introduce a 'mono-diet' for a few days. A mono-diet is a diet whereby at each meal only one kind of food is eaten. For example, for three days one could eat the famous soup diet, or one day only apples or green beans. As soon as the desired weight has been reached, one can stop eating mono-diets and only eat them again when the weight goes up. Always eat slowly and chew your food well.

People who want to lose weight should eat no bread, no refined carbohydrates or refined fat, no margarine or other industrial products. You will find further advice in *10 Golden Rules for Good Health*. Plenty of movement and exercise is one of the most important prerequisites for losing weight!

CHAPTER NINE

Chronic Disease

What Does the Word 'Disease' Really Mean?

Basically, disease or illness is nothing but the effort the organism makes when trying to detoxify and eliminate dangerous toxins, poisons and germs.

Every day, night, minute, second and fraction of a second such defensive reactions take place in our body. This wonderful defence system, which is already a part of every living organism before birth, will always react when we are threatened by even the smallest danger. For this purpose our body is provided with very complicated and extensive defence mechanisms.

As many of these protective defensive reactions take place deep down in our body, usually we do not notice them at all. We are so used to some of these reactions that we take no notice of them and accept them as being completely normal. For example, when something gets into our eyes, they will start watering. Coughing and sneezing are often defensive reactions against tiny particles of dust which threaten our respiratory tract.

We understand such defensive reactions and do not worry about them. As long as there are not too many pollutants or germs threatening our health everything will go smoothly. However, if one day the danger increases these defensive reactions will also become much stronger and as we do not understand their purpose any longer, we become frightened. From this moment on, we call such reactions, which are still nothing else but defensive actions of the organism, 'illness' or 'disease'.

All natural healing measures of the body are meant to destroy and eliminate toxins, dangerous germs and unusable substances which threaten the normal functions of the organism. Consequently there can be pain, fever and inflammation, which for us are the symptoms of a disease.

Usually every chronic disease starts with a rather simple acute health problem. Somewhere in the body, many toxins will have been accumulating, perhaps for a long time, until they impede normal body functions. Then the organism will intervene and the first defensive reactions in order to neutralise and eliminate these toxins will start. It goes without saying that the development of any illness is due to many different causes, like genetic factors, mental and emotional problems, social conditions, the climate, the constitution of the person concerned and much more.

In order to understand why chronic diseases have increased to such a frightening degree in the last 60 or 70 years, one has to realise that a combination of some of the following factors can be the cause of the chronic diseases of our time. These are, for example:

1. Harmful germs or other pathogen agents.
2. Genetic factors and defence mechanisms of the body.
3. Dangerous toxins.
4. Disease-provoking influences.

How to Change an Acute Illness into a Chronic Illness

An acute illness can become a chronic illness if the mistakes in living and eating habits which are usually the most important cause of illness are continued. In that case the organism will be inundated over and over again with the same kind of toxins and unusable substances so that the defence system of the body is overtaxed all the time.

Chronic disease will develop even sooner if the acute symptoms of illness (like fever, inflammation, headaches and so on) are suppressed by unsuitable measures. These paralyse the defence mechanisms of the organism and toxins cannot be excreted, and so travel deeper and deeper into the body tissues. After such a suppressive treatment the organism does not have enough strength left to defend itself and after some time there will be no further defensive reactions and the symptoms will disappear. Although the person in question will still feel quite tired, they will probably believe that they have been cured and will take up the same living and eating habits again without even suspecting that this is a great mistake.

From now on many toxins will again start accumulating. This goes on and on until the inner pollution has reached a certain level. Then for the second time the body will start taking defensive measures and often these reactions will take place somewhere else in the body. This apparently has nothing to do with the first reaction and will usually be considered to be a 'new disease', although the causes are still the same.

This pattern will continue until the body's defence mechanisms are so weak that for a long time no more defence reactions are possible. Now the disease becomes chronic. Every time that the organism has recovered somewhat, there will again be some weak or stronger defensive reactions, which right away will be suppressed by highly effective strong medication.

In such a way chronic illness is not only established, but is also nursed and tended in the best possible way to allow it to continue, sometimes for many years until the patient dies from innumerable side effects.

The Different Stages of Disease

Priessnitz, the most famous 'water doctor' of the past, used to say:

> Every substance which enters the human body through digestion or the skin, which the body cannot assimilate completely, is a poison. And the tremendous efforts the body makes in order to excrete toxins or germs, that possibly could harm the body, are the symptoms of an acute illness. If an acute illness is suppressed by medication, the original hostile [toxic] substances, which the organism wanted to get rid of, can in that case not be excreted; that is how chronic diseases develop.

And about medicine Priessnitz wrote the following: 'It is called poison when it is given to do harm, it is called medicine when it is given to cure.'

Those statements made by Priessnitz more then 150 years ago hit the nail right on the head and have been acknowledged not only by laymen but also by many reputable and famous physicians and scientists, like Dr

Lahman, Prof. Kotschau, Dr Bircher-Benner, Prof. Kollath, Prof. Bier, Alex Carrell, Paavo Airola, Ivan Illich and many others. Even Hippocrates said: 'A disease does not come out of the blue, it develops slowly because of daily sins against nature. When this happens often, toxins accumulate and illness breaks out.'

According to Priessnitz, illness develops in three different stages. During the first stage the body continuously tries to destroy and excrete harmful toxins and germs. When this first stage is suppressed by medication, the second stage starts and this is already chronic. Very often during this stage there are times of apparent wellbeing. At this stage recovery is rare. The organism can only keep harmful substances at a status quo. The patient does not generally feel well. He or she is in a state of 'semi-illness'; he is neither ill nor healthy. (In our time this is a very common situation, but people tend to regard this as 'normal'). The third stage, according to Priessnitz, is the stage of destruction. I quote: 'In this third stage the body has no more power and juices to tame the hostile substances within. The terrible suffering at this stage can only be provoked either by medicine or by a daily poisonous diet.'

Priessnitz, who treated and cured thousands of patients many years ago, was far ahead of his time in his knowledge and convictions. In 1952, after many years of research, his theories were not only confirmed by the brilliant physician and scientist Hans-Heinrich Reckeweg, but also scientifically proved. Unfortunately this has been completely ignored by modern medical science, as such ideas do not fit into the dogmatic pattern of our time, on the basis of which the entire industry of medical products and appliances has been set up.

For the pharmaceutical industry Reckeweg was a

spoilsport because he had the nerve, as a consequence of his research and practical experience, to condemn the suppression of symptoms as being, in most cases, dangerous and irresponsible. He suggested a complete reorientation of medical approaches and ways of treatment. However his proposal was rejected.

Reckeweg defined the development of chronic disease on the base of acute symptoms in an even more detailed way than Priessnitz. According to him chronic diseases develop in six different stages. I quote: 'All diseases are a sign of defensive measures which are taken by the organism against all substances which could harm or cannot be processed by the organism.' These substances act in the human body like poisons and Reckeweg called them 'homotoxins'. All diseases serve to render harmless, to excrete or encapsulate such toxins and therefore they are the expression of biologically effective and protective reactions.

The Development of Chronic Disease in Six Different Stages According to Dr Reckeweg

1. The first stage is the stage of excretion. At this stage the organism tries day and night to detoxify and excrete all harmful substances. Most of the time we hardly notice this. The excretion is done by way of the intestines, the urethra, the bladder, the skin, the mouth, the nose, the ears and the vagina and harmful substances leave the body through the stool, the urine, perspiration, saliva, semen, ear wax and so on.
2. The second stage is the stage of stronger reactions. Now the organism breaks up and dilutes all hard,

solid and tough substances so that they can be disposed of. Generally this is only possible with the help of fever and/or inflammation. During such a time the person in question usually feels quite ill; he may get the flu, a sore throat, inflammation of the tonsils, and many other health problems.

3. The third stage is the stage of the deposit of benign substances which cannot be excreted. They will be stored somewhere in the body and thereby diseases like gout, or gall bladder, kidney or bladder stones, different kinds of rheumatism, arteriosclerosis or arthritis in the initial stage can develop. We can also observe that as we grow older more unusable substances are deposited on the skin (age spots, warts etc). We should not forget that the skin changes we notice are only a fraction of the changes that take place in the inner skin, the mucous membrane.

These first three stages are still reversible; this means that the health problems and diseases which happen during these stages can still be cured or lessened when the person in question changes his or her lifestyle and ways of eating and is treated with natural remedies.

4. The fourth stage is the stage whereby toxins which have not been eliminated and could not be detoxified get deeper into the organism where they destroy cells, tissues and organs. This mainly happens after the symptoms of the previous stages of disease have been suppressed by unnatural means. Every simple health problem can in this way be changed into a lifelong chronic disease. This is the stage of impregnation.

5. The fifth stage is the stage of degeneration. In this

stage the 'homotoxins' have already destroyed so much of the organism that the illness might only be somewhat alleviated, as healing is usually no longer possible. Diseases like leukaemia, some kinds of cancer, multiple sclerosis, and some other diseases of the nervous system belong to this stage.

6. The sixth stage is the last stage, the so-called neoplasm stage. Now not only cells and tissues are destroyed, but also the assimilation of oxygen becomes quite impossible; enzymes are damaged and the normal body procedures can no longer take place. In this completely contaminated inner environment cancer cells can cause great damage and it is the end stage of many serious diseases.

To quote Dr Reckeweg: 'The more intensively and frequently the first three stages are suppressed, the more rapidly the next three stages will develop and sometimes the disease overlaps a stage and goes directly into the fifth or sixth stage.'

Of course not only wrong eating and living habits and environmental influences cause illness; mental influences also play an important role in the development of any disease. Today it is known that positive or negative thoughts can strengthen or weaken our natural immune system and our defences.

Dr Reckeweg has proved all the above-mentioned facts scientifically. Many physicians who are not influenced by dogmatic teachings and who still understand how necessary it is to be able to think logically and independently will understand the greatness of Dr Reckeweg's ideas.

Unfortunately, often in medicine financial and other interests are involved and there are still many fanatics in positions of power in medical circles, as well as in the pharmaceutical industry; therefore usually financial aspects have their first consideration. Business comes first! Most of these people will not even take the trouble to read, let alone think about, Dr Reckeweg's proposals. However there always were and still are physicians and scientists who agree with his ideas and who prefer real progress instead of dogmatism. One thing is sure: we cannot continue in this way, as it will be the end of health for millions of people.

FURTHER EXPLANATIONS
Because of inadequate nutrition and a wrong lifestyle the human body is constantly overloaded by more toxins. The body tries to excrete them and thus the first reactions to clean the body begin.

Some of the first simple symptoms may be the following: sniffles; angina; coughing; *fluor albis* (leucorrhoea, thrush, white vaginal discharge); vomiting; headache; diarrhoea; minor skin problems; itching; rashes.

If these symptoms are violently suppressed by medication and are not allowed to heal by themselves, more serious reactions start, such as flu; tonsillitis; bronchitis; gastrointestinal inflammations; migraine; constipation; eczema, acne or other skin problems; inflammation of the bladder; temperatures; fever.

If these problems are suppressed again and have no chance of healing on their own, there may be different reactions. The organism may not have enough strength to excrete the toxins and in this case they will deposited or accumulate somewhere in the body, for example as: nose polyps or mucous membrane polyps; kidney or gall bladder stones; uric acid deposits, which cause many rheumatic diseases; cysts (e.g. ovarian cysts); calluses, boils etc; oedemas; warts; age spots.

If the body still has the strength to excrete some of the toxins, the following diseases may develop: appendicitis; neuralgia (inflammation of the nerves); serious bronchitis, pneumonia or asthma; rheumatism of the muscles; inflammation of the kidneys; stomach ulcers; duodenal ulcers; diseases of the prostate; diseases of the ovaries; rhinitis; sinusitis etc.

If in the fourth phase of the illness the symptoms are suppressed by strong medication, most of the previous symptoms will become chronic or new diseases will develop such as myomas; osteoporosis; serious skin diseases; paralytic symptoms and paralysis; cirrhosis of the kidneys; sterility or impotence; tuberculosis in its various kinds; bone diseases; multiple sclerosis; syringomyelia; diseases of the blood.

In the following phase various cancerous and other degenerative diseases may develop. Thus if one doesn't stop the mistakes that were made in one's nutrition and lifestyle, step by step the diseases become more serious. Diseases do not always appear in this strict order, sometimes one or even several steps are skipped over and in an intermediate phase totally different diseases develop until they finally reach the incurable stage. This survey, then, is only an example for what eventually might happen. It would be impossible to list all the diseases that are known up to the present time systematically.

Chronic Civilisation Diseases

Chronic diseases are the greatest health problems of our time. Hospitals, clinics, old peoples' and nursing homes are full of sick people. Many of them will remain ill and will need constant care for the rest of their lives.

Statistics of the W.H.O. (World Health Organisation) show that since 1950 heart and circulation diseases have increased 18 times, rheumatic diseases 22 times, obesity 44 times, diabetes 70 times, multiple sclerosis 74 times, allergies 87 times and Alzheimer's disease 114 times. One can also add dental diseases, skin diseases, certain kinds of cancer, depression, mental diseases etc. Most of these diseases were known in ancient times. But in those days they were the exception to the rule and not, like nowadays, the ailments of millions of people. Only because 'progress' has made the production of innumerable food additives and the use of strong chemicals possible, could all the so-called 'civilisation diseases' increase at such a frightening speed.

Nowadays, dangerous infectious diseases are found mainly in tropical countries, where certain germs can cause life-threatening illness. Whether, in our moderate climate, such germs can settle and multiply depends on different factors. The well-known clinical encyclopaedia *Pschyrembel* says that: 'facultative pathological germs can only survive when the patient's well-being is reduced'. This means that in Western countries, only in the body of a patient whose defence mechanisms are weak could potentially dangerous germs cause illness.

However, this book is not about infectious diseases. It is about chronic modern diseases, which have but little to do with germs or 'pathogen agents'. Although they only seldom play a part in cases of the diseases of Western society, there is always a chance that bacteria and other harmful germs will multiply in a sick body. All living creatures, including germs, can live and propagate only when the environment and the food is right for them.

The kind of germs that might threaten our health feel at home in a polluted environment. Patients suffering from chronic diseases whereby the digestive tract, the inner environment, as it is called, is often very toxic, can be host to many dangerous germs that can trigger serious inflammations, although these germs are never the cause of the disease.

Whenever an infection is really life-threatening, most physicians will immediately kill the pathogen agents with strong medication and this can be lifesaving. Sometimes in the case of normal diseases this kind of treatment can be worse than the disease itself. The prescription of antibiotics or other strong medicine is at least partly responsible for the increase of all our civilisation, diseases, especially when this kind of medication is not really needed. It seems to be inexplicable, shocking and intolerable that a physician, who should be interested exclusively in our well-being, can make such terrible mistakes.

However, usually it is not the physician who is to blame, because he or she does not know any better. Most physicians are the victims of inadequate and faulty medical training at universities which are in many respects dependent on the dictates of a disease-oriented industry.

Because of misinformation during their studies, modern physicians are but seldom able to treat their patient's disease in the right way, as they do not even understand what the word 'disease' really means.

CHAPTER TEN

Staying Healthy While Getting Older

Getting Older

In our society when we think about getting older, very often this seems identical to us to getting ill. This is a completely wrong attitude.

What happens when we get older? Some people lose their hair and others do not; some people get many wrinkles, others many fewer; some people lose their teeth while others do not. Many people suffer from rheumatic diseases, but far from everybody. The list is endless and everyone gets old in his or her own way. Ageing cannot be prevented, but one can prevent illness.

Every cell in our body is a biological entity, which can stay healthy only when receiving quantitatively as well as qualitatively the right nutrients and when it can get rid of waste materials. The human being is also a biological entity which is subject to the same natural laws as the body cells. As long as someone is still young the assimilation of nutrients and the excretion of unusable substances usually functions all right. This changes when people become older. Getting older begins when the organism can no longer excrete all toxins, and these, depending on the living habits and the constitution of the person in question, accumulate somewhere in the body. When only few toxins accumulate, the elderly person usually stays quite healthy.

WHAT CAN WE DO TO PREVENT AN ACCUMULATION OF TOXINS?

When growing older one should eat less and stick to the right eating habits. It is very important not to eat anything between meals. One should get used to eating simple and healthy food. Elderly people should always remember to drink enough water. No black tea or coffee with cookies!

Having a regular bowel movement, urinating enough and perspiring every day guarantees the excretion of toxins. Regular exercise, like going for a walk, swimming, dancing or working in the garden will keep the body young and healthy. Light, air and sunshine are important. The human body needs contact with the forces of nature.

If, when one is still young, the excretion of toxins does not function well any more, this is a sign that there is an accumulation of too many toxins somewhere in the body. It indicates that the time has come to remedy the mistakes in one's eating and living habits and to clean the organism. A short fast, a change of diet, enemas, perspiring regularly, more sleep or a relaxing vacation could solve many problems.

If we do not feel well, we need a physician who knows about healthy nutritional and biological healing measures. After the right diagnosis, which will bring to light the fundamental causes of the illness, the physician can then help us to recuperate. We may need the following treatments: irrigation of the colon or enemas;

fasting; hydrotherapy; cupping; the Baunscheldt therapy; cantharidal plasters; neural therapy; homeopathy; or phytotherapy. Above all we need the right kind of nutrition, adjusted to our personal taste.

Natural Remedies

The following natural remedies are particularly suitable for treating elderly people.

HOMEOPATHY

Among the natural remedies, homeopathic remedies are clearly at the top. About 200 years ago Samuel Hahnemann established the law of 'similia similibus curentur' – the law of similitude – (disorders can be cured with substances which behave in a similar way). Homeopathic medicine still functions according to the following principles.

When a poison (or toxin) is causing certain symptoms, the same poison, but very highly diluted, can be used to cure these symptoms. Homeopathic medicine is prepared according to very exact rules. When a certain substance is highly diluted it loses it viciousness and on the contrary becomes a remedy with excellent healing properties.

The study of the so-called classical homeopathy is just as demanding as a university studies. A qualified and experienced homeopath can sometimes cure serious chronic diseases when traditional medicine can do nothing any more. Homeopathic medicine can always be recommended, especially for children and elderly people. Homeopathic remedies, when used in the right way, never can do any harm and can cure many ills.

Esoteric and other 'soft treatments'

As a reaction against too much materialism in our time and as a result of the loss of trust in traditional medicine, more and more people are becoming interested in esoteric and other so-called 'soft treatments'. These include aromatherapy, Dr Bach's flower remedies, meditation, massage, Ayurvedic medicine, light therapy, colour therapy, yoga, kinesiology and so on.

Many of these methods originally came from China, India and the Arabian countries, as well as from the Incas, the Indians and primitive tribes. Often these methods of healing were, and still are, very valuable. As long as these healing methods can support the healing of physical and mental problems, and as long as the person in question does not concentrate too much on his or her own problems and disease, these methods are very beneficial.

However, it is hardly ever possible to cure a serious chronic disease of our Western world with these therapies. These healing ways originally came from the East or from parts of the world where living conditions and eating habits were and sometimes still are completely different and usually much healthier and more natural than in our countries. Some of these methods are really wonderful and with their help people can sometimes restore their lost physical or mental equilibrium. However, as long as the organism of the person in question is still being inundated with the toxins of the Western world, there will often be a relapse. Only when the organism has been cleaned on all levels and no more toxins are supplied will the above-mentioned healing methods really make sense.

There are many thousands of people who think that only by meditating or using other soft healing measures can they cure disease. Thereby they often waste much time and money, because some unscrupulous fashionable gurus and other persons exploit sick people who believe in them. It makes absolutely no sense to try to heal the mind when the body is still full of toxins and unusable substances.

A meaningful life, which includes work, hobbies, enough exercise, friends and if possible a loving partner, are important prerequisites for a healthy life, especially as one grows older. If one is really ill, healing is only possible if the patient has enough intelligence to understand that the way towards recovery demands sacrifice and is not always easy. It may be necessary to give up many habits one has grown fond of, and it is also very important to really wish to get well again.

Our health does not depend on preventative medicine and medical care, or on fate. At least two-thirds of all chronic diseases we can prevent ourselves. Most of the time we can decide ourselves if during the last ten or twenty years of our life we will stay healthy, or if we will spent these years on crutches, in a wheelchair or in bed.

CHAPTER ELEVEN

Alzheimer's Disease

Alzheimer's Disease Seen in a Different Light

As we approach the end of this book, I think it is very important to say something about one of the most feared diseases of western civilisation. Alzheimer's disease is one of several such diseases for which medicine could do so much more. Now, an estimated 100 million people worldwide are suffering from this terrible disease and by the year 2030 their number will be about 160 million. Alzheimer's is the third greatest cause of death in most industrial countries, behind cancer and heart disease.

Many millions of pounds are spent on research to find the causes of Alzheimer's and this disease has become a real goldmine for the pharmaceutical industry, Patients are given the latest drugs against the symptoms of the disease and as the need arises, physicians will also prescribe tranquillisers or stimulants.

As long as the patient, to some extent, is still responsive, counselling and psychotherapy will be tried and through occupational therapy his or her memory and other brain functions will be stimulated. But how long is it still possible to train a diseased brain, which becomes more and more uncommunicative and dysfunctional?

The cause of Alzheimer's is still a mystery and there is no known cure. At present the most important goal for the pharmaceutical companies is to develop a drug which may delay or even stop the further development of the disease. During research, more abnormalities are found in the brains of diseased patients all the time. Researchers try to find out what substances or agents are responsible for the destruction of brain cells and the formation of plaques (explained further below). Based on their discoveries many drugs have been developed and over and over again we hear a song of praise for some new medicine. And always there is great disappointment as in practice these drugs either turn out to be useless or have such dangerous side effects that they are soon taken off the market again.

A Hypothesis

Nature does not do anything without a reason and many changes that take place in the brain of Alzheimer patients and which we call abnormal, could in fact be very normal defensive reactions. When scientists look at the brain of diseased Alzheimer's patients, one of the most noticeable things is the formation of plaques, which form a kind of coating or crust.

In nature, the formation of crusts is quite normal. Whenever there is an open wound, the body will cover it up as soon as possible. A crust serves as protection, so that no further toxins can enter the wound and the underlying connective tissue can heal. In order to form such a hard or soft crust many enzymes, white blood cells, as well as different body juices and other known and also still unknown helpers will be employed and the procedure is always more or less the same. At first different enzymes will be released from the damaged cells and these break down proteins, which are split up in order to build such a protective crust.

Of course, in the brain the same thing can also happen. Why should reactions in the brain be different from reactions that happen in other parts of our body? As in nature, everything always happens according to the same natural laws, so the formation of plaques indicates that parts of the brain which have somehow been damaged are now being covered by a protective layer.

Although the brain is one of the best-defended regions of the human body, its defensive mechanisms are not able to fight against the steadily increasing number of unnatural toxins in our environment. In a healthy body the defensive mechanisms do not permit the entry of toxic material into the brain, for normally this is prevented by the 'brain barrier' (or blood barrier), the goalkeeper which is situated at the base of the brain. When this protective barrier becomes porous and breaks down as a consequence of our contaminated environment, more and more poisonous toxins can enter our brain, while damaging millions of nerve cells. In that case the brain will counteract by covering the wounded places with plaques in order to protect the rest of the brain. The human body will produce and provide anything needed for the construction of these plaques. Most abnormal enzymes, or other deviations from the norm that scientists discover, are probably needed simply as construction materials. If science tries to destroy the plaques which are only one part of an exactly programmed recovery programme, this will be only a waste of time and money. Such measures have nothing to do with the original cause of the disease.

NATURE ALWAYS WINS

Maybe some day science will succeed in developing new drugs which will inhibit the work of abnormal enzymes or other agents, and the formation of plaques will be prevented or interrupted. However, nature has very definite intentions when constructing these plaques and within a very short time our body will find other, more cunning, means to produce other kinds of plaques or similar crusts.

It would be far better to find out why this protection is needed. It is certainly not abnormal that such plaques develop, but the damage done previously to the brain is abnormal, and it is our task to find out how and why this happens and what the real culprit is.

Wrong Diagnosis and Senseless Treatments

How little we understand about natural connections shows clearly when we use anti-inflammatory drugs to treat Alzheimer's patients.

An inflammation, like a fever, as we learned in chapter six, is a normal reaction of the body's own defence system. When health and the normal functioning of the organism are threatened, fever and inflammation are emergency measures by which more damage is prevented.

Most anti-inflammatory remedies are very toxic and have many side-effects. The same is true of other strong medication from pharmaceutical companies which is used to kill bacteria and other micro-organisms. As dangerous bacteria and other germs can only thrive and multiply in a polluted environment, this means that such micro-organisms are never the original cause of any disease. Although micro-organisms may play a secondary role in Alzheimer's, we can rule them out as the original cause, and killing them with toxic drugs is only a symptomatic treatment, which raises the level of toxicity in the organism of the patient even more.

Abnormal calcium deposits in the brains of patients are sometimes seen as a cause of Alzheimer's. However, we should realise that this is merely a consequence of the disease. It is known that when tissues are damaged, as for example in inflammatory rheumatic and other diseases, calcium deposits are formed. These deposits prevent further harm and are a protective measure. In the case of Alzheimer's disease, it seems logical that calcium deposits in some parts of the brain are nothing more than a protective measure the brain takes in order to prevent further damage.

A Hereditary Disposition and the Wrong Genes?

'Bad' genes which cause a specific disease most certainly have not always been present in certain families. If this were so, there would be no more people left on earth, as all of them would have died long ago as a consequence of hereditary diseases. Like everything else in nature such genes could develop and prevail as a consequence of the living conditions of a certain era. Probably these genes could develop properly only when people did not have an intact defence mechanism.

Genes have a shorter or longer survival rate depending on their environment. Some genes probably can survive for five, ten or twenty human generations; others may exist for much longer. During each susequent generation the influence of most genes become a little weaker. This explains why in every era of the history of humankind different kinds of diseases have occurred, depending on the ever-changing environment.

All the changes that take place in our body cells are intimately connected with the genes in those cells. So-called 'bad' genes, which are the cause of specific diseases, influence all functions within their host cells. If these 'bad' or abnormal genes were destroyed or exchanged, all the living conditions in the host cell would be topsy-turvy and nobody knows what could happen. The development of specific genes depends on many different factors. Anyone who believes that it is possible to destroy or exchange certain genes without problems is rather naive.

MULTIPLE CAUSES

Like the other diseases prevalent in western society, Alzheimer's disease always has multiple causes. As yet it is not known, and maybe it will never be known, which combination of environmental influences, toxins, harmful substances, mental problems, wrong eating habits and a wrong lifestyle or a lack of vital substances play a role in the development of this terrible disease.

Modern industry now uses more than 100,000 man-made chemicals, which do not exist in nature. Natural chemicals, which in nature exist only in combination with countless other substances, are taken out of their relationship with other substances and are then concentrated. These chemical substances then become mavericks and they will paralyse all the normal defence reactions of the organism. Most of these chemicals have not even been tested for neurological effects.

The best-known and most often used man-made chemicals are prescription drugs and also many over-the-counter remedies. How in the world is it possible that such medicaments, which will always increase the amount of toxins in the human body, are used for Alzheimer's patients!

Many food additives are also toxic. When the same kind of food is eaten often, the safety margins are exceeded and as the human being is a creature of habit, this happens all the time. Other poisons originate in the body itself, particularly in the intestinal tract, where for example chronic constipation can cause much spoilage and toxicity.

PRIONS

Prions are extremely small parts of rogue proteins which, according to some scientists, come from our intestinal tract. It may be quite possible that these prions then pass into the blood and the brain, by way of the brain barrier if some part of this barrier has been damaged.

Prions may develop when animals have been fed ruminant waste products (see *10 Golden Rules for Good Health*). When cows eat the vegetarian food which is natural to them and which they can assimilate and digest, they are healthy because in that case their meat consists of normal proteins. However, when cows are treated like carnivorous animals and are fed meat products, even if those products stem from healthy animals, these cannot be completely digested as nature has not foreseen this. Although such cows still grow, their defence system weakens and they need more and more medication. The proteins of the meat from cows fed on food that is unnatural to them cannot be normal, and could be very toxic for humans. Prions are known to cause different diseases, especially mental ones, and they could also be one of the most important causes of Alzheimer's disease. In this respect science at last is following some logical conclusions.

WRONG EATING AND LIVING HABITS

Day by day, mainly by way of the bloodstream, a constant flow of information and building material reaches our brain and more than 60 per cent of the nutrients which come from food are used by the brain. The function and the health of our brain depends mainly on the kind and the quality of the food we eat. Alzheimer's is a disease of modern society, which like all such diseases is closely connected with our polluted environment and wrong eating and living habits. Such habits are often due to poor education, poverty and environmental problems.

DANGEROUS RADIATION

More radiation than we have ever known before is now a part of our modern lifestyle and not only X-rays or high-voltage radiation, like radar aerials, but also, as is now known in certain scientific circles, regular exposure to extremely low radiation could be dangerous for our health. The dangerous effects of radiation, especially in diseases of the brain like Alzheimer's, should be taken very seriously indeed. Knowledge about these dangers is still in its infancy.

OTHER CAUSES

Of course, many of the other factors associated with our modern life mentioned in this book may be responsible for the development and the frightening increase of this disease, for example smoking, drugs, poverty, poor diet and the lack of specific vital nutrients, and much more. All these things cause a weak defence system and are often prerequisites for the development of serious illness.

The human brain uses up at least one third of all the nutrients and vital substances supplied by our nutrition every day. Therefore it is indispensable to immediately stop the influx of any harmful substances, like alcohol, nicotine, coffee, additives and so on and to prescribe a very simple and healthy diet for all Alzheimer's patients. Unfortunately in most clinics and care centres these people are still given coffee, tea and many industrially refined foods. Even smoking is still permitted in many of these places!

Anyone who complains about the fact that all this will need far too much time, work and money should try to think about the time, the work and the money that is wasted during a long chronic illness. As long as these patients are served food and drinks which are lacking in many vital substances and are, on the contrary, harmful, we cannot expect any progress. This has to be changed, as otherwise there will always be more disease and unspeakable suffering.

OLD AND NEW WISDOM
The primary cause of many diseases of our time is pollution. Some pollution comes from outside the body and some originates in our own intestines. Hippocrates and his successors were absolutely sure that in the case of diseases of the brain, the whole person is invariably ill. Freud too believed that some day we would find a physical cause for such diseases.

In the treatment of Alzheimer's disease and other diseases of civilisation there is no progress, because medicine is mainly interested in suppressing the symptoms. As long as the body is still inundated with toxins any of the acclaimed so-called progress in the research and treatment of Alzheimer's will be a dead end. Instead of constantly mistaking the symptoms for the cause of the disease and wasting enormous amounts of money, much positive help could be given, and for only a fraction of the money spent.

While studying the methods of treatment and achievements of the old physicians and the work of some of the courageous physicians of our time, it should be clear what should be done. In the case of Alzheimer's especially, cleaning methods and special treatments used in the past, combined with new knowledge about vital substances like vitamins and minerals etc, and modern treatments like neural therapy, acupuncture, cranial treatment, magnet therapy and many other old and new healing ways could bring amazing results.

'Healing is cleaning' was always one of the most important and very strict rules of successful physicians of the past. It is extremely important to clean the organism on all levels, as is explained in this book. Many of the formerly used derivative and excretory measures can produce real miracles and the physician who has the courage to really make use of these will be amazed at his or her success.

With the help of modern diagnostic methods it is possible by examining the blood, the urine and the hair to find out which harmful substances or toxins are contaminating the organism and if there is a lack of certain vitamins, minerals and other vital substances.

It is high time to stop the prevailing dogmatism; one should overcome all prejudices and only do what is right for the patient. It really is a shame when an intelligent physician believes that nothing can be done for these patients. The most important thing is therefore to find the right physician, one who has enough courage and who will take the trouble to really help his or her patients. More and more is now known about the healing methods of olden times and it is unforgivable not to use this knowledge when treating Alzheimer's and other supposedly 'incurable' diseases.

Epilogue

In the course of time there have been many different opinions about what causes disease and it is interesting to observe that after some deviations the general opinion of well-known physicians always came back to the original ideas of Hippocrates.

In the earliest times disease was considered as a punishment from the gods, and evil spirits, poisons and harmful substances that spoiled the body juices were also held responsible for all diseases.

Most Greek physicians from Kos, as well as from Knidos, were convinced that unhealthy nutrition in a qualitative and quantitative sense, and wrong behaviour, like gluttony, excessive drinking and an immoral lifestyle could make people ill. Hippocrates himself said that a surplus of food, fat, blood and residues of metabolic processes, which could not be excreted from the body, endangered health.

Paracelsus (1493–1541) said: 'Where pain is, toxins have accumulated.' He also thought that poor metabolism, abnormal residues and the accumulation of surplus body juices could cause disease and he warned people about the dangers of suppression of habitual secretions, like perspiration, menstruation and bleeding piles. For many physicians of olden times, diseases were due to the wrong composition of body juices, especially the blood, in a quantitative and qualitative sense and to the accumulation of many toxins.

Then, in the nineteenth century, Louis Pasteur and Robert Virchow changed the entire image of medicine. Louis Pasteur had proved that dangerous germs caused all our diseases and Robert Virchow claimed that our state of health depended mostly on the condition of our body cells.

From this time on, the governing majority of orthodox medicine, in collaboration with the pharmaceutical industry, declared all previous knowledge antiquated. Therefore medical education at the different universities followed once again the example of the school of Knidos, concentrating mainly on the suppression of symptoms. Orthodox medicine not only came to a standstill, but modern diseases increased in a frightening way and in our time people are suffering more and more from chronic diseases.

However, running parallel to and as a reaction to this health-endangering attitude, an ever-stronger movement has started in favour of a more humane and natural kind of medicine. In this book I have told you of many possible causes of disease and have also provided information about some new ideas which it would be worthwhile to follow up.

The belief of primitive people that disease was a punishment of the gods is extremely interesting. There is a profound truth in this. Nowadays people who destroy their environment and who sin against the laws of nature are punished by droughts, floods and other natural disasters and those who change wonderful natural food into artificial products are punished by the appearance of new and terrible diseases, which our medical establishment does not know how to cure.

As Dr Alfred Vogel said so often in his lectures, 'In nature everything is in balance. Man has put it out of balance, but still nature will always try to bring harmony.'

Index